MCQs in
Human Anatomy

MCQs in Human Anatomy

Dr. D.K. Chopade
M.B.B.S., M.S.
Grant Medical College and
J.J. Hospital, Byculla, Mumbai-400008
Ph. : 022-3704190 / 3735555, 0253-342082
Email : drchopade@hotmail.com, drchopade@yahoo.com
Web : http://usa.internations.net/health/drdkc

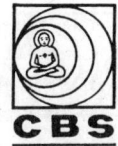

CBS PUBLISHERS & DISTRIBUTORS PVT. LTD.
New Delhi • Bangalore • Pune • Cochin • Chennai (India)

ISBN : 81-239-0870-9

First Edition : 2003
Reprint : 2004, 2005, 2006, 2007, 2009, 2011

Copyright © Publisher

All rights reserved. No part of this book may be reproduced or transmitted in any form or by any means, electronic or mechanical, including photocopying, recording, or any information storage and retrieval system without permission, in writing, from the publisher.

Published by Satish Kumar Jain and produced by V.K. Jain for
CBS Publishers & Distributors Pvt. Ltd.,
CBS Plaza, 4819/XI Prahlad Street, 24 Ansari Road, Daryaganj,
New Delhi - 110002, India.   • Website: www.cbspd.com
e-mail: delhi@cbspd.com, cbspubs@vsnl.com, cbspubs@airtelmail.in
Ph.: 23289259, 23266861, 23266867   • Fax: 011-23243014

Branches:
- **Bengaluru:** Seema House, 2975, 17th Cross, K.R. Road, Bansankari 2nd Stage, Bengaluru - 560070   Ph.: +91-80-26771678/79   Fax: +91-80-26771680   • E-mail: cbsbng@gmail.com, bangalore@cbspd.com
- **Pune:** Bhuruk Prestige, Sr. No. 52/12/2+1+3/2, Narhe, Haveli (Near Katraj-Dehu Road By-pass), Pune - 411051   Ph.: +91-20-64704058/59, 32342277   • E-mail: pune@cbspd.com
- **Kochi:** 36/14, Kalluvilakam, Lissie Hospital Road, Kochi - 682018, Kerala • Ph.: +91-484-4059061-65   Fax: +91-484-4059065   • E-mail: cochin@cbspd.com
- **Chennai:** 20, West Park Road, Shenoy Nagar, Chennai - 600030   Ph.: +91-44-26260666, 26208620   • Fax: +91-44-42032115   E-mail: chennai@cbspd.com

Printed at :
J.S. Offset Printers, Delhi

Preface

Multiple Choice Questions are used for assessment of students in all universities as well as various competitive and entrance examinations in the medical field all over the world.

Multiple Choice Questions form an integral part of any evaluation system because of their inherent objective nature and validity. In this book, a sincere attempt is made to prepare the MCQs in simple and clear language with clearly defined problems keeping in mind their validity. Questions of all difficulty levels (I, II & III) are included for all types of students. Examples of all the types of MCQs are given in the chapter 'Introduction to MCQ's', but only single best response types MCQ's are prepared, as these are the most preferred type. More than 2000 MCQ's are included in this book. For the convenience of students the questions are arranged regionwise under the heads as General Anatomy, Embryology, Genetics, Radiology and Imaging, Upper Limb, Lower Limb, Thorax, Abdomen, Pelvis and Perineum, Head, Face, Neck and Nervous System and special senses. Questions on Histology are covered in all the regions.

I hope, that the book will inspire the students to learn Human Anatomy intensively in retrospect and provide students an opportunity to assess themselves the depth of their knowledge. This book will also be of immense help during practical examinations. I am sure that these MCQs will stimulate the students to further enrich their knowledge from the textbooks.

Constructive suggestions from the readers will be appreciated for further improvements.

Dr. D.K. Chopade

Acknowledgements

In writing this book I have been greatly influenced by my former Head of the Department and teacher Prof. Dr. S.M. Sant who has guided and continuously encouraged me. Without his guidance it would have been difficult to make this a good quality MCQ book of this standard. I am benefitted by helpful suggestions on the book from Prof. Dr. G.J. Khadse, Head, Deptt. of Radiology of J.J. Hospital. I am greatly indebted to them.

My many thanks are due to my colleagues Dr. Rajan Wable and Dr. Mandar Ambike for their help in reading the proof and giving valuable suggestions. I am grateful to all my students who inspired me for writing this book. I cannot forget Mr. Baliram Surse for his generous help in typing the MCQs. I am grateful to all my colleagues, friends and teachers who have assisted me from time to time.

Finally, I would like to dedicate this book to my wife Sandhya and son Sandesh for their forbearance and continued goodwill.

8 October, 2001   D.K. Chopade

Contents

Preface v
Acknowledgements vi

- I. Introduction to MCQs 1
  1. Structure of MCQs 1
  2. Types of MCQs 2
  3. How MCQs are marked 4
  4. Suggestions for solving MCQs 4
  5. Techniques of solving MCQs 5
- II. Embryology 6
- III. Genetics 31
- IV. General Anatomy 39
- V. Upper Limb 56
- VI. Lower Limb 75
- VII. Thorax 100
- VIII. Abdomen, Pelvis and Perineum 103
- IX. Head, Face, Neck and Nervous System 133
- X. Special Senses 185
- XI. Radiology and Imaging Methods 196

Answers 201
References 211
Format of Model MCQ Answer Sheet 213

Chapter I

Introduction to Multiple Choice Questions

Throughout the world Multiple Choice questions, generally called as MCQs are used for the objective assessment of students knowledge at various university as well as medical entrance examinations. MCQs are easy and accurate to mark and are very reliable.

1. Structure of MCQs
Individual MCQs are also known as items. The various components of MCQs are as follows :
  a) *Direction :* These are instructions given to the candidates about the nature of the questions and for solving them.
  b) *Problem :* It is the stem or base of the MCQ. It is the problem to be solved depending on the types of MCQ. In single best response type it may be an incomplete statement to be completed or a direct question to be answered.
  c) *Choices :* These are four or five suggested answers for the problem. These are also known as alternatives. The correct choice (answer) is called as a key and others as the distractors.

2. Types of MCQs
There are various types of MCQs. But the most widely and commonly used is single best response type.

1. Single best response type
In this type of MCQ usually four choices are given out of which only one is the correct answer, and other three are the distractors. These MCQs test recall of the facts, reasoning and thinking abilities of the examinee.

Directions : Each of the following question is followed by four alternatives. Choose the most appropriate answer and cross (x) the box of the corresponding alphabet.

Subtypes of single best response MCQs
  (i) Single completion type
  (ii) Question type
  (iii) Negative form type

(i) Single completion type

Example : Parasympathetic grey column is confined to the spinal cord segments :
    a) third cervical to first thoracic
    b) second thoracic to first lumber
    c) ninth thoracic to first lumber
    d) second to fourth sacral
Answer : (a) ☐ (b) ☒ (c) ☐ (d) ☐

(ii) Question type

Example : Which of the following tracts provides the route for the spinovisual reflexes?
    a) spinorubral
    b) spinothalamic
    c) spinotectal
    d) spinoreticular
Answer : (a) ☐ (b) ☒ (c) ☐ (d) ☐

(iii) Negative form type

Example : All of the following parts of the large intestine show the presence of the mesentery except :
    a) appendix
    b) transverse colon
    c) rectum
    d) sigmoid colon
Answer : (a) ☐ (b) ☒ (c) ☐ (d) ☐

2. Multiple completion type

Directions : One or more of alternatives given are correct for each of the following questions. Cross the alphabet box corresponding to the correct answer as per the code given below :
    a) If only 1, 2 are correct
    b) If only 2, 4 are correct
    c) If only 1, 2, 3 are correct
    d) If only 4 is correct

Example : Anterior relations of right kidney include :
    1. stomach
    2. liver
    3. body of pancreas
    4. duodenum
Answer : (a) ☐ (b) ☒ (c) ☐ (d) ☐

3. Multiple true false type :

Directions : Please respond by crossing T (True) or F (False) to each of the four alternatives bearing in mind that all, some or none of the alternatives may be true :

Example : Pertaining to the mesonephric duct :

a) In males, it forms the epididymis, vas deference and ejaculatory ducts
b) In females, it forms uterus, uterine tubes and cervix
c) Ureteric diverticulum originates from its caudal end
d) It is also known as Mullerian duct

Answer : (a) ☐ (b) ☒ (c) ☐ (d) ☐

4. Relationship Analysis Type/Assertion Reason Type :

Directions : Each question given below consists of two statements. Statement 1 (Assertion) and Statement 2 (Reason) connected by the term because. Cross the appropriate box corresponding to the answer using the code given below :
  a) If both statements are true and statement 2 is a correct explanation of statement 1
  b) If both statements are true and statement 2 is not a correct explanation of statement 1
  c) If statement 1 is true and statement 2 is false
  d) If statement 1 is false and statement 2 is true
  e) If both statements are false

Example :
Statement 1 : Visceral pleura is not sensitive to pain
Statement 2 : Visceral pleura is innervated only by the autonomic nerves

Answer : (a) ☐ (b) ☒ (c) ☐ (d) ☐

5. Matching type

Directions : Each question given below consists of four/five lettered headings followed by a list of numbered words or phrases. Select one lettered heading that is most closely related to the numbered words. Each of heading can be used once, more than once or not at all in the set.

a) inguinal canal   1. obturator nerve
b) femoral canal   2. lymph node
c) carpel tunnel   3. femoral nerve
d) adductor canal   4. spermatic cord
e) mandibular canal   5. median nerve
                           6. inferior alveolar nerve

Answer : (a) ☐ (b) ☒ (c) ☐ (d) ☐

6. Pictorial type :

Direction : For each of the following statements described select the diagram of the most appropriate anatomical location :
  1. It is known as palleopallium
  2. It is involved in the auditory pathway
  3. It transmits projection fibers
  4. It forms the lateral wall of third ventricle

Answer : (a) ☐ (b) ☒ (c) ☐ (d) ☐

7. Case history type :

Example : A 10-year-old girl presented with complaints of severe headache and diplopia after an accident. On examination a convergent squint is observed. Which of the following nerve is most likely to be affected?
    a) oculomotor
    b) trochlear
    c) ophthalmic
    d) abducent
    Answer : (a) ☐ (b) ☒ (c) ☐ (d) ☐

3. How MCQs are marked?

There are two ways of marking the MCQs.
  a) *Positive marking* : Most of the university examination systems use positive marking pattern for MCQs. In this pattern the correct answer is given half or one or more than one marks. For an incorrect answer (response) no mark or zero mark is given. Students are advised to solve all the MCQs, even those they do not know at all. Luck factor is said to play a role in positive marking system.
  b) *Negative marking* : In this system, marks are deducted from the total correct score for an incorrect answer. Marks to be deducted for one incorrect answer varies from place to place, but usually half mark is deducted when one mark is given for a correct answer. This pattern discourages the students from random guessing.

Appropriate marking of the answer in the box provided is very important. If possible, students should become familiar with the appropriate answer sheet for MCQs. Commonly used format of the answer sheet is provided at the end of this book for the ready reference.

4. Suggestions for solving MCQs :

  a) The most common type of MCQs asked are the single best response. It is very important to practice the MCQs of the type expected in the examination. Practice should be made of using different techniques of solving the questions, marking the answers correctly and appropriately on the expected format of answer sheet and answering the questions within the limited time.
  b) During examinations, before attempting any answers, read the question paper carefully. MCQs that the candidate is sure about should be answered first. Remember that first thoughts are often the best. As far as possible do not make changes in answers once marked. Remaining questions can then be solved by using different techniques and making semi-informed guesses.
  c) In examinations adopting positive marking pattern, solve all the questions, including those you are not sure about. But, do not go for random guessing in the negative marking pattern examinations.

5. Techniques of Answering MCQs

You can achieve the best possible result in the MCQ examination, if your approach towards answering the MCQs is systematic. You can do this by practising different techniques to answer the questions :
a) *Ideal technique :* Immediately after reading the question, if the answer strikes in your mind, go through the choices and select the one.
b) *Common technique :* Most of the times you are familiar with the stem, but are not sure about its answer or do not know it. If you go through the choices, you can recognise its answer.
c) *Extraction technique :* You are not familiar with the stem, but are familiar with at least three of the choices and are sure that these can not be the correct answers. Select the fourth choice as a correct answer.
d) *Elimination technique :* Using the common sense to select one option as a correct answer by eliminating three options as incorrect ones when you are not familiar with the stem as well as options.
e) *Random guess technique :* When you can not use any of the above methods, go for random guess. This is advisable only in examinations adopting positive marking pattern.

Chapter II

EMBRYOLOGY

1. Embryo is the developing individual during which of the following periods?
   a) during first seven days after fertilization
   b) during first two months after fertilization
   c) from third month until birth
   d) from fertilization until birth

2. The chromosomal constitution of the spermatids is
   a) 46 XY
   b) 23 XY
   c) 23 X or 23 Y
   d) none of the above

3. Which of the following defines spermiogenesis?
   a) formation of sperms from spermatogonia
   b) formation of sperms from spermatids
   c) nourishment of sperms
   d) abnormal sperm formation

4. When 'Y' bearing sperm fertilizes an ovum, the offspring is
   a) a male
   b) a female
   c) a hermophrodite
   d) any of the above

5. Which of the following statements regarding oogenesis is **incorrect**?
   a) first polar body contains 46XX chromosomes
   b) second polar body contains 23X chromosomes
   c) second polar body is formed at the time of fertilization
   d) one primary oocyte forms only from one ovum

6. Acrosomal cap of the sperm is formed by
   a) mitochordria
   b) nucleus
   c) endoplamic reticulum
   d) golgi apparatus

7. Annulus of the middle piece of sperm is formed by
   a) mitochondria
   b) centriole
   c) Golgi apparatus
   d) smooth endoplasmic reticulum

8. Sheath of middle piece of sperm is formed by
   a) mitochondria
   b) centriole
   c) Golgi apparatus
   d) nucleus

9. Which of the following leads to the formation of a triploid zygote?
   a) failure of extrusion of second polar body
   b) nondisjunction
   c) anaphase lag
   d) none of the above

10. Which of the following phenomena describes amphimixis?
    a) associated with the fusion of male and female gamete nuclei
    b) which ensue upon the entry of the spermatozoon in the ovum
    c) concerned with the transformation of spermatid into the sperum
    d) by which a mature ovum forms an embryo without fertilization

11. Totipotency of early blastomeres can be described as
    a) organ specificity of blastomere
    b) each of the blastomere can form any type of tissue
    c) each of the blastomere is capable of forming an individual
    d) none of the above

12. The usual site of zygote implantation in the uterus is
    a) posterior wall near the cervix
    b) posterior wall near the fundus
    c) anterior wall near the cervix
    d) anterior wall near the fundus

13. Termination of the ectopic pregnancy usually occurs by
    a) fundamental nutritive problem of the embryo
    b) endocrine insufficiency
    c) an immune maternal response
    d) a mechanical or vascular accident

14. The term 'Placenta praevia' means implantation of zygote
    a) at any place inside or outside the uterus
    b) at normal site
    c) near the internal os
    d) near the fallopian tube

15. All of the following statements regarding the pro-chordal plate are correct **except**
    a) it forms the oropharyngeal membrane
    b) the notochord extends upto its cephalic margin
    c) it contributes to the general head mesenchyme
    d) endoderm of the yolk sac is thickened and attached firmly to the overlying ectoderm

16. Plane of bilateral symmetry of the embryo is established
    a) as soon as the bilaminar disc is formed
    b) only after the formation of the pro-chordal plate
    c) only after the formation of the notochord
    d) only after the formation of the neural tube

17. Primitive knot is formed at the
    a) caudal end of the prochordal plate
    b) caudal end of the primitive streak
    c) cephalic end of the primitive streak
    d) cephalic end of the cloacal membrane

18. Which of the following forms the notochord?
    a) the prochordal membrane
    b) the cloacal membrane
    c) the primitive streak
    d) the primitive knot
19. The caudal end of the neural groove in the early embryo is located at
    a) the primitive knot
    b) the caudal end of the primitive streak
    c) the cranial end of the cloacal membrance
    d) none of the above
20. In the embryo with the neuroentric canal, a transerve section across the embryo cranial to the primitive knot shows that the roof of the yolk sac in the median plane is formed by
    a) the endoderm
    b) the ectoderm
    c) the notochordal cells
    d) neural plate
21. Which of the following is the source of the intraembryonic mesoderm?
    a) primitive streak
    b) notochord
    c) neural crest
    d) all of the above
22. Which of the following is probably involved in the inductive process of cranial structures?
    a) notochord
    b) primitive knot
    c) prochordal membrane
    d) none of the above
23. Septum transversum is formed by
    a) cardiogenic intraembryonic mesoderm
    b) non-cardiogenic intraembryonic mesoderm
    c) extraembryonic mesoderm in front of cardiogenic mesoderm
    d) junction of cardiogenic and extraembryonic mesoderm
24. The process of neural tube formation is initiated in the
    a) cranial most end of neural groove
    b) upper cervical region
    c) thoracic region
    d) caudal end of neural groove
25. Which of the following statements regarding the choroid plexuses is incorrect?
    a) formed only in the thin parts of the primary cerebral vesicles
    b) present only in the walls of the ventricular cavities
    c) formed in all the primary cerebral vesicles
    d) forms the cerebrospinal fluid
26. Which of the following statement/s regarding the tela choroidea is/are correct?
    a) It is the fold of pia mater covering the ependyma.
    b) It is formed in the thin parts of primary brain vesicle.
    c) Along with the capillary fringes it forms the choroid plexus.
    d) all of the above

27. Which of the following structures is **not** formed by the primitive embryonic ectoderm?
    a) dermis of the skin
    b) anterior lobe of hypophysis cerebri
    c) enamel of teeth
    d) the chromaffin organs
28. Which of the following is formed by the ectoderm?
    a) epithelium lining the auditory tube
    b) epithelium of the thyroid and parathyroid glands
    c) the plain muscle of iris   d) dermis of skin
29. All of the following structures are formed by the primitive embryonic ectoderm **except**
    a) the epidermis and appendages of skin
    b) neuroepithelium of eyeball
    b) the lens of eyeball   d) dermis of the skin
30. The epithelium of prostate is formed by
    a) ectoderm   b) endoderm
    c) mesoderm   d) all of the above
31. Which of the following parts of teeth is **not** formed by the intraembryonic mesoderm?
    a) pulp   b) dentine
    c) enamel   d) all of the above
32. The cortex of the suprarenal gland is derived from
    a) the mesoderm   b) the neural crest cells
    c) the endoderm   d) the surface ectoderm
33. Suprarenal medulla is derived from
    a) the mesoderm   b) the endoderm
    c) the surface ectoderm   d) the neural crest cells
34. All of the following structures are derived from the neural crest cells **except**
    a) adrenal cortex   b) sympathetic ganglia
    c) parasympathetic ganglia   d) dorsal root ganglia
35. Which of the following tissues of the epithelial character are derived from the mesoderm?
    a) endothelium of blood vessels   b) mesothelium
    c) synovial membranes   d) all of the above
36. The linning of anterior chamber of eye is derived from
    a) neuroectoderm   b) surface ectoderm
    c) mesoderm   d) endoderm
37. Mesenchymal cells are derived from
    a) mesoderm   b) endoderm
    c) cytotrophoblast   d) all of the above

38. Myoepithelial cells of sweat, sebaceous and mammary glands are derived from
    a) general body ectoderm
    b) mesoderm
    c) neural crest
    d) all of the above

39. Which of the following cells is not derived from neural crest cells?
    a) oligodendrocytes
    b) astroytes
    c) microglia
    d) neurons

40. All of the following cells are derived from neural crest **except**
    a) tanycytes
    b) Schwann cells
    c) satellite cells of sensory ganglia
    d) odontoblasts

41. Cells belonging to the APUD (Amine Precursor Uptake and Decarboxylation) group include all of the following **except**
    a) pinealocytes
    b) magnocellular neurons of hypothalamus
    c) all retinal cells
    d) oligodendrocytes

42. Which of the following meninges is derived from the paraxial mesoderm?
    a) dura mater
    b) arachnoid mater
    c) pia mater
    d) all of the above

43. Primordial germ cells appear in the wall of the yolk sac during development at the end of the
    a) second week
    b) third week
    c) fourth week
    d) fifth week

44. The primordial germ cells pass from the yolk sac to developing gonads
    a) by way of blood
    b) as these are actively pulled by the developing gonads
    c) by ameboid movement
    d) yolk sac pushes it to the gonads

45. Primitive germ cells arrive in the developing gonads at
    a) the end of third week
    b) beginning of fourth week
    c) beginning of fifth week
    d) end of the fifth week

46. Ovarian follicular cells originate from
    a) primordial germ cells
    b) surface epithelium covering the ovary
    c) fibroblasts
    d) neural crest cells

47. The total number of germ cells in the ovary reaches its maximum
    a) by fifth month of development
    b) after birth
    c) by third week of development
    d) at puberty

48. A maximum number of oogonia appearing in the ovary during development is
    a) 7 million
    b) 7 billion
    c) 7 lac
    d) 7 thousands

49. Graafian follicle of the ovary is
   a) a primary oocyte with surrounding flat epithelial cells
   b) a primary oocyte with surrounding multiple layers of granulosa cells
   c) secondary oocyte with surrounding flat epithelial cells
   d) large ovarian follicle with antrum folliculi

50. Until puberty is reached, primary oocytes remain in which of the following phases of division?
   a) prophase of first meiosis
   b) metaphase of first meiosis
   c) prophase of second meiosis
   d) metaphase of second meiosis

51. The total number of primary oocytes at birth is
   a) 0.7. to 2 lacs
   b) 0.7 to 2 millions
   c) 0.7 to 2 thousands
   d) 7 to 20 million

52. The total number of oocytes ovulated in the reproductive lifetime of an individual are fewer than
   a) 5
   b) 50
   c) 500
   d) 5000

53. How many primordial follicles begin to mature with each ovarian cycle after puberty?
   a) 1 to 4
   b) 5 to 15
   c) 15 to 30
   d) 30 to 50

54. All of the following statements regarding the zona pellucida are true **except**
   a) it is a layer of glycoprotein on the surface of graafian follicle
   b) finger-like processes of follicular cells extend across it
   c) it allows transport of material from follicular cells to oocyte
   d) it dissolves in the uterine cavity before implantation of ovum.

55. At maturity the diameter of the graafian follicle may be
   a) 0.1 mm
   b) 1 mm
   c) 10 mm
   d) 100 mm

56. Which of the following statements describes the 'cumulus oophorus' in graafian follicle?
   a) cells covering the antrum folliculi
   b) cells covering the graafian follicle on outer aspect
   c) cells radiating from the ovum
   d) cells surrounding the ovum

57. With each ovarian cycle a number of follicles begin to develop but usually only one reaches its full maturity while others
   a) wait for next ovarian cycle
   b) degenerate and become atretic
   c) regress to primordial follicle
   d) become corpus luteum

58. A primary oocyte resumes its first meiotic division
    a) immediately after birth
    b) as soon as the follicle begins growing
    c) as soon as the follicle is mature
    d) as soon as it is fertilized

59. The polar body practically receives
    a) no nucleus
    b) no cytoplasm
    c) no nucleus and cytoplasm
    d) both nucleus and cytoplasm

60. The first polar body is located
    a) between zona pellucida and cell membrane of oocyte
    b) outside zona pellucida
    c) inside cell membrane of oocyte
    d) outside the theca

61. The second maturation division of the oocyte is completed
    a) shortly before ovulation
    b) immediately after ovulation
    c) only if the oocyte is fertilized
    d) just before fertilization

62. Which of the following statements is certain?
    a) first polar body undergoes a second division
    b) fertilized ovum is accompanied by three polar bodies
    c) second maturation division of oocyte is complete only if it is fertilized
    d) none of the above

63. Diameter of mature oocyte is
    a) 0.012 mm
    b) 0.12 mm
    c) 1.2 mm
    d) 12 mm

64. During growth of the ovarian follicle, the theca cells secrete
    a) oestrogen
    b) progesterone
    c) luteinizing hormone
    d) follicle stimulating hormone (FSH)

65. Corpus luteum secretes
    a) oestrogen
    b) progesterone
    c) luteinizing hormone
    d) follicle stimulating hormone (FSH)

66. In humans the fertilized oocyte reaches the uterine lumen in approximately
    a) 3 to 4 hours
    b) 7 hours
    c) 3-4 days
    d) 7 days

67. If fertilization fails to occur, after ovulation the corpus luteum reaches maximum development on
    a) third day
    b) sixth day
    c) ninth day
    d) fifteenth day

Chapter II

Embryology

68. 'Corpus luteum of pregnancy' continues to secrete progesterone until the end of
    a) fourth month
    b) fifth month
    c) fourth week
    d) fifth week

69. Fertilization occurs in
    a) ampullary region of uterine tube
    b) isthmus of uterine tube
    c) uterine cavity
    d) on the surface of ovary

70. If not fertilized, the oocyte is thought to die after ovulation within
    a) 6 to 12 hours
    b) 12 to 24 hours
    c) 24 to 48 hours
    d) 48 to 72 hours

71. Capacitation of sperm in the female reproductive tract lasts approximately
    a) 7 minutes
    b) 7 hours
    c) 7 days
    d) 7 seconds

72. Which of the following statements describe capacitation of sperm
    a) passage of sperm through the ejaculatory ducts
    b) removal of glycoprotein and seminal plasma proteins from the plasma membrane covering acrosomol region
    c) fusion of plasma membrane with the outer acrosomal membrane
    d) release of acrosomal contents

73. After deposition in female genital tract how many sperms reach the ovum?
    a) 3 to 5
    b) 30 to 50
    c) 300 to 500
    d) 3000 to 5000

74. Corona radiata cells of the ovum at fertilization are dispersed by
    a) combined action of sperm and tubal mucosa enzymes
    b) enzyme hyaluronidase
    c) contraction of fallopian tube
    d) none of the above

75. The permeability of zona pellucida changes
    a) when the head of sperm comes in contact with it
    b) when the head of sperm comes in contact with the oocyte surface
    c) when the sperm enters oocyte
    d) only after the completion of second meiotic division by ovum

76. In the human, at fertilization which of the following parts of sperm enter the cytoplarm of oocyte?
    a) only nucleus
    b) only head
    c) head and tail without plasma membrane
    d) head and tail with plasma membrane

77. When is the chromosomal sex of the embryo determined?
    a) even before fertilization
    b) at fertilization
    c) after 12 weeks of development
    d) at birth

78. Alteration in structure and composition of zona pellucida of ovum possibly through removal of specific receptor sites for sperms is known as
    a) activation
    b) capacitation
    c) zona reaction
    d) parthenogenesis
79. Which of the following parts of morula contribute to the embryo proper?
    a) outer cell mass
    b) inner cell mass
    c) both outer and inner cell mass
    d) none of the above
80. Disadvantage of in vitro fertilization technique is
    a) risk of producing malformed children is high
    b) risk of chromosomal abnormalities is high
    c) low success rate of the procedure
    d) preimplantation embryo is highly susceptible to teratogenic insult
81. Implantation of the embryo starts at about the
    a) third day
    b) fourth day
    c) fifth day
    d) sixth day
82. As per the estimations, what percentage of all pregnancies end in spontaneous abortions?
    a) 10%
    b) 25%
    c) 50%
    d) 75%
83. What percentage of all newborns have congenital defects?
    a) 0.2 to 0.3%
    b) 2 to 3%
    c) 3 to 5%
    d) 5 to 10%
84. In which stage of menstrual cycle the endometrium passes after 2 to 3 days of ovulation?
    a) menstrual phase
    b) proliferative phase
    c) secretary phase
    d) reparative phase
85. At the time of implantation of ovum, the mucosa of uterus is in
    a) secretary phase
    b) proliferative phase
    c) menstrual phase
    d) premenstrual phase
86. Which part of the endometrium is expelled during menstruation?
    a) only epithelium
    b) whole endometrium
    c) only spongy layer
    d) spongy and compact layer
87. All of the following statements regarding the cytotrophoblast are true **except**
    a) it is the inner layer of trophoblast
    b) it is a multinucleated zone without distinct cell boundaries
    c) mitotic figures are found in it
    d) thickness of cytotrophoblast does not increase considerably

Chapter II
Embryology

88. Uteroplacental circulation is established in
    a) second week
    b) third week
    c) fourth week
    d) fifth week
89. Which of the following is the chorionic cavity?
    a) yolk sac cavity
    b) amniotic cavity
    c) extraembryonic coelom
    d) intraembryonic coelom
90. Cellular columns of which of the following describe the primary villi?
    a) syncytotrophoblast
    b) cytotrophoblast covered by syncytotrophoblast
    c) cytotrophoblast containing the mesenchyme
    d) cytotrophoblast containing blood vessels
91. Which of the following describes the 'chorionic plate'?
    a) extraembryonic mesoderm lining the inside of cytotrophoblast
    b) cytotrophoblast covered by syncytotrophoblast
    c) extraembryonic mesoderm covering wall of yolk sac
    d) extraembryonic mesoderm covering amnion
92. What is recapitulation?
    a) During development, human embryo shows the structural features of the ancestors.
    b) Temporal variation in growth of the embryo.
    c) Spatial variation in growth of the embryo.
    d) Temporal and spatial variation in morphogenetic movement of embryo.
93. Gastrula represents
    a) monolaminar embryonic disc
    b) bilaminar embryonic disc
    c) trilaminar embryonic disc
    d) all of the above
94. Accretionary growth can be defined as an increase in the
    a) size of the specific individual cell
    b) number of cells
    c) amount of structural intercellular material
    d) nuclei and associated cytoplasm in syncytia
95. Which of the following represents the auxetic growth?
    a) increase in size of facial bones
    b) increase in size of the smooth muscle cells of pregnant uterus
    c) continual replacement of dead cells, as in epidermis
    d) all of the above
96. During development, all of the following structures change their positions due to differential growth rate in relation to the adjacent structures **except**
    a) gonads
    b) spinal cord
    c) kidneys
    d) eyes

97. A view that 'various organ primordia appearing during development are essentially new formations and are not present in the zygote' is known as
   a) preformation
   b) epigenesis
   c) total information content
   d) none of the above

98. Which of the following views describes 'preformation'?
   a) all the mature body structures are present in the zygote
   b) organ primordia appearing during development are new formations
   c) both nucleus and cytoplasm direct the formation of new structures
   d) all of the above

99. Continual replacement of dead cells as in epithelia represents what type of growth?
   a) accretionary
   b) multiplicative
   c) auxetic
   d) none of the above

100. Differentiation can be defined as
   a) ability of the cells to form any type of body tissue
   b) reversible cell changes in reponse to environment
   c) irreversible, inheritable differences between cells
   d) none of the above

101. A 'luxury molecule' in a cell during embryonic develpment is
   a) synthesized by cell for its viability
   b) unique molecule synthesized or inherited for its differentiation
   c) molecule taken up by the cells from the extracellular compartment
   d) none of the above

102. All of the following structures are formed by the mesoderm **except**
   a) gonocytes in both sexes
   b) prostatic utricle
   c) vesical trigone
   d) adrenal cortex

103. Which of the following represents the rudimentary homologue of uterus in male?
   a) appendix of testis
   b) appendix of epididymis
   c) prostatic utricle
   d) vesical trigone

104. Which of the following muscles show obvious migration of its myotome during development?
   a) limb muscles
   b) intercostal muscles
   c) tongue muscles
   d) abdominothroacic diaphragm

105. Which of the following shows late appearance of the loci of the red blood cell formation?
   a) red bone marrow
   b) liver
   c) spleen
   d) yolk sac mesenchyme

106. All of the following epithelia are endodermal in origin **except**
   a) parotid gland epithelium
   b) oesophageal epithelium
   c) respiratory epithelium
   d) pancreatic epithelium

107. Which of the following epithelia is derived from the mesoderm?
    a) oral epithelium
    b) respiratory epithelium
    c) digestive epithelium
    d) uroepithelium
108. Caudal limit of hindgut endoderm is
    a) anorectal junction
    b) the level of anal valves
    c) the lower end of anal canal
    d) junction of sigmoid colon and rectum
109. Somites are the blocks of which of the mesoderm?
    a) paraxial
    b) intermediate
    c) lateral plate
    d) extraembryonic
110. Segmentation of paraaxial mesoderm begins in the embryo at the beginning of
    a) fourth week
    b) fifth week
    c) sixth week
    d) seventh week
111. Segmentation of paraxial mesoderm is initiated near the
    a) lower cervical region
    b) region of hindbrain
    c) caudal end of the neural tube
    d) cranial most end of neural tube
112. Maximum number of somites formed in embryo is
    a) 30-32
    b) 32-34
    c) 38-40
    d) 42-45
113. All of the following statements regarding the somites are true **except**
    a) these are formed in the intermediate mesoderm
    b) in all 42-45 pairs of somites are formed
    c) its first occipital pair is asymmetrical
    d) a typical somite contains a transient central cavity
114. All of the following tissues in the wall of the digestive tract are formed by the splanchnopleuric mesoderm **except**
    a) serosa or adventitia
    b) smooth muscles
    c) submucosal connective tissue
    d) lining epithelium
115. Mesoderm covering the amnion is continuous with which of the following mesoderm?
    a) extraembryonic splanchnopleuric
    b) intraembryonic
    c) extraembryonic chorionic
    d) all of the above
116. The amount of liquor amni in the amniotic cavity at the end of pregnancy is usually about
    a) 0.1 litre
    b) 0.5 litre
    c) 1 litre
    d) 2 litres
117. A condition is called as hydramnios when the amniotic fluid in the amniotic cavity is
    a) about less than 500 ml
    b) about one litre
    c) between one to two litres
    d) more than 2 litres

118. Oligohydramnios is associated with
    a) oesophageal atresia
    b) anencephaly
    c) open spina bifida
    d) agensis of kidneys
119. Hydramnios is associated with
    a) open spina bifida
    b) agenesis of kidney
    c) atresia of lower urinary tract
    d) low birth weight babies
120. Normal umbilical hernia of the midgut in the embryo develops between
    a) third to sixth week
    b) sixth to tenth week
    c) tenth to fifteenth week
    d) fifteenth to twentieth week
121. The umbilical cord contains all of the following structures after tenth week **except**
    a) yolk sac
    b) allantoic duct
    c) vitelline and allantoic vessels
    d) extraembryonic coelomic sac
122. The yolk sac and its duct contained in umbilical cord usually disappears
    a) at the end of first trimester
    b) by the midpregnancy
    c) at the end of 7th month of pregnancy
    d) at full term
123. When fully developed, on an average the length of umbilical cord is
    a) 5 cm
    b) 50 cm
    c) 100 cm
    d) 500 cm
124. The maternal surface of basal plate of the placenta shows
    a) mesodermal layer
    b) synctotrophoblastic layer
    c) cytotrophoblastic cells
    d) fetal blood vessels
125. In relation to the menstrual phase of uterus, when does the ovulation occur?
    a) at the beginning of menstrual phase
    b) at the end of menstrual phase
    c) about 14 days before the next menstrual flow
    d) at any time during menstrual cycle
126. 'Decidua capsularis' is the part of decidua
    a) between the conceptus and the uterine cavity
    b) between the conceptus and uterine muscular wall
    c) which lines the remainder of the body of uterus
    d) which forms placenta
127. Placenta is subsequently developed in which of the following parts of decidua?
    a) parietalis
    b) capsularis
    c) basilis
    d) any of the above
128. The 'decidua parietalis' and capsularis are in contact by the beginning of which month of pregnancy?
    a) third
    b) fifth
    c) seventh
    d) ninth

129. All of the following terms define the human placenta **except**
    a) bidiscoidal
    b) haemochorial
    c) labyrinthine
    d) chorioallantoic
130. The expelled full term placenta has an average weight of
    a) 50 gm
    b) 100 gm
    c) 500 gm
    d) 1000 gm
131. The chorionic plate of the placenta is covered on its fetal aspect by
    a) syncytium
    b) cytotrophoblast
    c) connective tissue layer
    d) amniotic epithelium
132. Leucocytes are more numerous in the blood of the umbilical vein than in that of the umbilical artery suggesting that
    a) more leucocytes are formed in umbilical vein
    b) more leucocytes are destroyed in umbilical artery
    c) leucocytes migrate from the maternal to fetal blood
    d) leucocytes migrate from fetal to maternal blood
133. Which of the following describes placenta accreta?
    a) exceptional adherence to the decidua basalis
    b) placenta adherent to myometrium
    c) invasion by placental tissue completely through the uterine wall
    d) margins of the placenta are undercut by a deep groove
134. When the fetal umbilical cord is attached between the centre and margins of the placenta, then the placenta is known as
    a) battledore
    b) succenturiate
    c) praevia
    d) increta
135. Placenta invading the complete uterine wall is known as placenta
    a) increta
    b) percreta
    c) praevia
    d) battledore
136. Placenta overlying the internal os of uterus is known as placenta
    a) battledore
    b) increta
    c) praevia
    d) percreta
137. Twinning occurs in about every
    a) 80 births
    b) 180 births
    c) 500 births
    d) 800 births
138. Which of the following is most common combinations of twins?
    a) boy-boy
    b) girl-girl
    c) girl-boy
    d) all are equally common
139. All of the following statements regarding the dizygotic twins are true **except**
    a) they result from two separate ova
    b) each embryo develops in its own chorionic sac
    c) the twins are of different genetic constitution
    d) they bear greater resemblance to one another than other siblings

140. All of the following statements regarding the monozygotic twins are true **except**
    a) they arise from a single ovum fertilized by two sperms
    b) the twins may share one chorionic sac
    c) the twins are always of the same sex
    d) monozygotic twinning is a hereditary character
141. Irregular meiotic cycle during oogenesis may lead to
    a) monozygotic twinning
    b) dizygotic twinning
    c) uniovular but dispermic twinning
    d) any of the above
142. In fetal life the notochord forms
    a) vertebral bodies
    b) complete intervertebral discs
    c) annulus fibrosus of intervertebral disc
    d) nucleus pulposus of intervertebral disc
143. Notochordal cells in the nucleus pulposus commence to degenerate
    a) after six months of fetal life
    b) six months after birth
    c) six years after birth
    d) after second decade of life
144. All of the following bones are described as dermal bones **except**
    a) sphenoid
    b) frontal
    c) parietal
    d) squamous part of temporal
145. Immediately after head fold formation, the stomatodeum is bounded caudally by
    a) forebrain
    b) septum transversum
    c) cardiac prominance
    d) mandible
146. Which of the following arches is named as 'hyoid arch'?
    a) first
    b) second
    c) third
    d) fourth
147. Musculature derived from the third pharyngeal arch is supplied by which of the following nerves?
    a) mandibular
    b) glossopharyngeal
    c) facial
    d) superior laryngeal
148. Nerve supply to which of the following phanyngeal arches is uncertain?
    a) third
    b) fourth
    c) fifth
    d) sixth
149. The nasolacrimal duct is formed by
    a) craniopharyngeal canal
    b) nasopalatine canal
    c) stomatodeal fissure
    d) nasomaxillary groove
150. In which of the following cogenital anomaly, the nasolacrimal duct persists as an open furrow?
    a) lateral cleft lip
    b) median cleft lip
    c) facial cleft
    d) cleft nose

Chapter II

151. Which of the following structures contributes to the external acoustic meatus?
    a) first pharyngeal groove
    b) first pharyngeal pouch
    c) first branchial arch
    d) all of the above
152. When present, branchial cysts lined by stratified squamous spithelium are derived from
    a) placodal vesicles associated with vagus and glossopharyngeal nerves
    b) persistant remnant of pharyngeal pouches
    c) second branchial cleft
    d) cervical sinus
153. All of the following structures are the derivatives of first pharyngeal arch **except**
    a) incus
    b) malleus
    c) spine of sphenoid
    d) sphenomandibular ligment
154. All of the following are the derivatives of the second pharyngeal arch **except**
    a) stapes
    b) styloid process
    c) stylomandibular ligament
    d) lesser cornu of hyoid
155. Which of the following is the derivative of the sixth pharyngeal arch?
    a) lower body of hyoid bone
    b) cricoid cartilage
    c) arytenoid cartilage
    d) thyroid cartilage
156. In all pharyngeal arches the aortic arch is caudomedial and the nerve is rostromedial to the cartilage **except**
    a) first arch
    b) fourth arch
    c) second arch
    d) sixth arch
157. All of the following muscles are derived from the first pharyngeal arch **except**
    a) tensor palatini
    b) levator palatini
    c) tensor tympani
    d) mylohyoid
158. All of the following muscles are derived from the hyoid arch **except**
    a) occipitofrontalis
    b) stylohyoid
    c) anterior belly of digastric
    d) stapedius
159. Which of the following muscles is derived from third pharyngeal arch?
    a) styloglossus
    b) stapedius
    c) stylohyoid
    d) stylopharyngeus
160. Pre-trematic nerve to the first pharyngeal arch is regarded as branch of
    a) trigeminal
    b) facial
    c) glosssopharyngeal
    d) vagus
161. Ultimobranchial body gives rise to
    a) parafollicular cells of thyroid
    b) follicular cells of thyroid
    c) parathyroid gland
    d) thymus

162. All of the following muscles are derived from the mesoderm of upper limb bud **except**
    a) lattissimus dorsi
    b) trapezius
    c) levator scapulae
    d) pectoralis major

163. Which of the following muscles exhibit active migration during development from its origional place?
    a) deltoid
    b) pectoralis major
    c) lattissimus dorsi
    d) supraspinatus

164. All of the following statements regarding the development of upper limb are correct **except**
    a) by the eighth week of development, it attains the foetal position
    b) it rotates laterally in subsequent development
    c) its preaxial border becomes medial
    d) its ventral surface becomes anterior

165. Premature closure of sagital suture of skull results in
    a) scaphocephaly
    b) acrocephaly
    c) plagiocephaly
    d) microcephaly

166. Acrocephaly results from premature closure of
    a) sagittal suture
    b) coronal suture
    c) coronal and lambdoid sutures on one side
    d) all the sutures

167. In the newborn, when extremities are represented only by hands and feet attached to the trunk by small irregular bone; the condition is known as
    a) amelia
    b) micromelia
    c) meromelia
    d) polymelia

168. Period of organogenesis during intrauterine development is
    a) first four weeks
    b) fourth to eighth weeks
    c) eighth to twelfth weeks
    d) twelfth weeks till birth

169. All of the following are derived from ectoderm **except**
    a) muscles of iris
    b) myoepithelial cells of mammary gland
    c) myoepithelial cells of sweat glands
    d) muscles of middle ear

170. Preotic somites give rise to
    a) preauricular muscles
    b) muscles of tongue
    c) extraocular muscles
    d) muscles of iris

171. Muscles of tongue are derived from
    a) pre-otic somites
    b) occipital somites
    c) pharyngeal arch mesenchyme
    d) splanchnic mesoderm

172. Which of the following glands is derived from the endoderm?
    a) pancreas
    b) mammary gland
    c) adrenal gland
    d) sweat gland

Embryology

173. Which of the following parts of skin is derived from dermatome?
    a) epidermis
    b) dendritic cells
    c) dermis
    d) sebaceous glands
174. Enlargement of breast in male is known as
    a) polymastia
    b) gynaecomastia
    c) macromastia
    d) amastia
175. "Palatine tonsil" is derived from
    a) first pharyngeal cleft
    b) second pharyngeal cleft
    c) first pharyngeal pouch
    d) second pharyngeal pouch
176. Endoderm of third pharyngeal pouch gives rise to
    a) superior parathyroid gland
    b) inferior parathyroid gland
    c) thyroid gland
    d) tonsil
177. Epithelium of which of the following parts of oral cavity is derived from endoderm?
    a) inner aspect of lips and cheeks
    b) gums
    c) tongue
    d) palate
178. Posterior one third of the tongue is derived from
    a) hypobranchial eminence
    b) copula
    c) tuberculum impar
    d) lingual swellings
179. The downgrowth of thyroglossal duct appears between
    a) two lingual swellings
    b) lingual swellings and tuberculum impar
    c) tuberculum impar and copula
    d) copula and the dorsal part of hypobranchial eminance
180. Artery of midgut is
    a) superior mesentric
    b) coeliac
    c) inferior mesentric
    d) hepatic
181. All of the following are the derivatives of the foregut **except**
    a) thyroid gland
    b) pancreas
    c) liver
    d) spleen
182. Post-arterial segment of the midgut loop proximal to the caecal bud gives rise to
    a) proximal part of ileum
    b) terminal part of ileum
    c) caecum
    d) ascending colon
183. Viewed from the ventral side the midgut loop exhibits rotation of
    a) 90 degree anticlockwise
    b) 90 degree clockwise
    c) 270 degree anticlockwise
    d) 270 degree clockwise
184. The skin of the philtrum of the lip is derived from which of the following processes?
    a) frontonasal
    b) lateral nasal
    c) maxillary
    d) mandibular

185. Congenital megacolon results from
    a) abnormal thickness of muscular wall of colon
    b) atresia of colon
    c) non-development of nerve plexures in the wall of colon
    d) imperforate anus
186. Which of the following conditions is associated with imperforate anus?
    a) incomplete septation of cloaca
    b) congenital megacolon
    c) tracheoesophageal fistula
    d) pyloric stenosis
187. Non-return of congenital umbilical hernia is known as
    a) exomphalos
    b) volvulus
    c) diverticulum ilei
    d) umbilical sinus
188. All of the following structures are developed from the mesenchyme of septum transversum **except**
    a) bile capillaries
    b) hepatic sinusoids
    c) capsule of liver
    d) connective tissue of liver
189. The hepatic bud grows from the endoderm at the summit of
    a) upper and lower half of foregut
    b) foregut and midgut
    c) midgut and hindgut
    d) upper and lower half of hindgut
190. All of the following statements regarding the ventral pancreatic bud are correct **except**
    a) it arises in the angle between hepatic bud and the duodenum
    b) it migrates towards dorsal pancreas
    c) it forms head and uncinate process of pancreas
    d) its duct system forms accessory pancreatic duct
191. The amount of blood circulating through the lungs in the foetal life is rich enough to provide adequate oxygen for sustaining life at its earliest by which month?
    a) third
    b) fifth
    c) seventh
    d) ninth
192. Which of the following laryngeal abnormalities is known as laryngoptosis?
    a) larynx abnormaly low in neck
    b) abnormaly large laryngeal saccule
    c) duplicated larynx
    d) cogenital atresia of larynx
193. The mesodermal cells lining the intraembryonic coelom gives rise to
    a) epithelium
    b) endothelium
    c) mesothelium
    d) all of the above
194. The infracardiac bursa is derived from the
    a) right pneumoenteric recess
    b) left pneumoenteric recess
    c) pleural cavities
    d) pericardial cavity

195. All of the following contributes to the development of lesser sac **except**
    a) right pneumoenteric recess   b) peritoneal cavity
    c) greater omentum   d) left pneumoenteric recess
196. All of the following structures contribute to the development of diaphragm **except**
    a) pleuroperitoneal membranes   b) mesentries of stomach
    c) septum transversum   d) body wall mesoderm
197. Which of the following is the first organ in the fetus to start functioning
    a) heart   b) kidney
    c) brain   d) liver
198. Which of the following structures contributes to the formation of inferior vena cava?
    a) sinus venosus   b) right vitelline vein
    c) right common cardinal vein   d) right umbilical vein
199. Left horn of sinus venosus contributes to the formation of
    a) left atrium   b) right atrium
    c) coronary sinus   d) inferior vena cava
200. All of the following layers are formed by myoepicardial mantle **except**
    a) parietal pericardium   b) epicardium
    c) myocardium   d) endocardium
201. The venous valves of sinu-atrial orifice gives rise to
    a) septum primum   b) septum secondum
    c) septum spurium   d) septum intermedium
202. In the adult anatomy, the limbus fossa ovalis represents lower free edge of
    a) septum primum   b) septum secundum
    c) septum spurium   d) septum intermedium
203. The septum intermedium is derived from
    a) the roof of atrial chamber   b) the atrioventricular cushion
    c) venous valves of sinoatrial orifice
    d) dorsal wall of atrial chamber
204. The right venous valve of sinuatrial opening contributes to all of the following **except**
    a) interatrial septum   b) crista terminalis
    c) valve of inferior vena cava   d) valve of coronary sinus
205. The left atrium is derived from all of the following **except**
    a) primitive atrial chamber   b) atrioventricular canal
    c) absorbed proximal parts of pulmonary veins
    d) sinus venosus
206. The pulmonary and aortic valves are derived from
    a) atrioventricular cushions   b) the endocardial cushions
    c) spiral septum   d) bulbar ridges

207. All of the following septa contribute to the development of definitive interventricular septum **except**
    a) spiral
    b) bulbar
    c) intermediate
    d) primitive interventricular
208. Which of the following interatrial septal defect may be associated with the defects of endocardial cushion?
    a) ostium primum defect
    b) ostium secondum defect
    c) patent foramen ovale
    d) all of the above
209. Fallot's tetralogy consists of all of the following defects **except**
    a) interventricular septal defect
    b) overriding aorta
    c) pulmonary stenosis
    d) hypertrophy of left ventricle
210. All of the following arch arteries disappear during development **except**
    a) first
    b) second
    c) third
    d) fifth
211. Which of the following arch arteries gives rise to ductus arteriosus?
    a) right sixth
    b) left sixth
    c) right fourth
    d) left fifth
212. Which of the following statements describes the fate of umbilical arteries?
    a) both disappear
    b) right disappears and left forms the ligamentum teres hepatis
    c) they contribute to the formation of inferior vena cava
    d) both the arteries remain as superior vesical arteries in their proximal part
213. Venous passage connecting the right hepatocardiac channel to the left umbilical vein is called as
    a) ductus caroticus
    b) ductus venosus
    c) ductus arteriosus
    d) oblique vein
214. Gonadal veins are remnants of
    a) subcardinal veins
    b) supracardinal veins
    c) posterior cardinal veins
    d) anterior cardinal veins
215. Ligamentum teres of the liver is the remnant of
    a) left umbilical artery
    b) left umbilical vein
    c) sinus venous
    d) sinus arteriosus
216. Oxygenated blood from the placenta comes to the fetus through
    a) umbilical artery
    b) vitelline artery
    c) umbilical vein
    d) vitelline vein
217. Which of the following parts of mesoderm plays an important role in the development of urogenital system?
    a) lateral plate somatopleuric
    b) lateral plate splanchnopleuric
    c) paraaxial
    d) intermediate

Embryology

218. During fetal development after the subdivision of cloaca, the mesonephric duct opening lies at the junction of
    a) vesicourethral canal and definitive urogenital sinus
    b) urinary bladder and primitive urethra
    c) pelvic and phallic part of definitive urogenital sinus
    d) allantois and cloaca
219. The developing kidney of man is called as
    a) pronephros
    b) mesonephros
    c) metanephros
    d) none of the above
220. All of the following statements regarding the human pronephros are correct **except**
    a) It is formed in relation to cervical region.
    b) It is functional in the early fetal development.
    c) It disappears soon after its formation.
    d) The nephric duct formed in relation to it persists.
221. Metanephros develops in which of the following region?
    a) sacral
    b) lumbar
    c) thoracic
    d) cervical
222. Which of the following structures of the adult kidneys are formed by the metanephric blastema?
    a) glomerulus
    b) excretory tubules
    c) collecting tubules
    d) calyceal system
223. The definitive renal artery represents
    a) the twelfth thoracic segmental branch of aorta
    b) second lumbar segmental branch of aorta
    c) fifth lumbar segmental branch of aorta
    d) lateral sacral artery
224. Before the rotation of the fetal kidney, its hilum faces
    a) anteriorly
    b) posteriorly
    c) medially
    d) laterally
225. 'Horseshoe kidney' is the anomaly of development of kidney in which
    a) the kidney remains lobulated
    b) two kidneys lie on one side, the adjacent poles being fused
    c) two kidneys form one mass lying in midline or on one side
    d) the lower poles of kidneys fuse by the connecting isthmus
226. Failure of excretory tubules of metanephros to establish contact with the collecting tubules leads to
    a) congenital polycystic kidney
    b) horseshoe kidney
    c) pancake kidney
    d) hydronephrosis
227. Which of the following structures of the urinary bladder develops from endoderm?
    a) whole epithelium except that of trigone
    b) epithelium of trigone
    c) muscular wall
    d) serosa

228. 'Ectopia vesicae' is a developmental anomaly of urinary bladder in which
   a) it communicates with the rectum
   b) it is duplicated
   c) it is divided into upper and lower compartments
   d) its cavity is exposed on the surface of body

229. Which part of the posterior wall of the male urethra is derived from mesoderm?
   a) prostatic part upto the opening of ejaculatory ducts
   b) prostatic part below the opening of ejaculatory ducts
   c) membranous part   d) spongy part

230. In female foetus, the genital tubercle gives rise to
   a) clitoris   b) labia minora
   c) labia majora   d) urethra

231. During gonadal development, spermatogonia and oogonia are derived from
   a) coelomic epithelium covering gonadal ridge
   b) mesenchymal cells of gonadal ridge
   c) yolk sac endoderm
   d) yolk sac mesoderm

232. Ductuli efferents of testis are derived from
   a) the mesonephric duct   b) paramesonephric duct
   c) remaining excretory mesonephric tubules
   d) primitive sex cord

233. The gonads acquire male or female morphological characteristics only after which week of development
   a) fifth   b) seventh
   c) ninth   d) twelfth

234. Which of the following chromosomal pattern is seen in the Klinefelter's syndrome?
   a) 47 XYY   b) 47 XXX
   c) 47 XXY   d) 45 XO

235. In pure gonadal dygenesis, the chromosomal pattern is
   a) 46 XX or 46 XY   b) 46 XX and 46 XY
   c) 47 XXY   d) 45 XO

236. In which of the following conditions primordial germ cells do not migrate to the gonad
   a) Turner's syndrome   b) Klinefelter's syndrome
   c) pure gonadal dysgenesis   d) true hermaphrodite

237. In testicular feminization syndrome the karyotype is
   a) 46 XY   b) 46 XX
   c) 46 XY/46XX   d) 47 XXY

Embryology

238. When genotypic sex is masked by phenotypic appearance the condition is known as
    a) true hermaphroditism
    b) pseudohermaphroditism
    c) gonadal dysgenesis
    d) Turner's syndrome
239. The most common cause of female psuedohermaphrodite is
    a) adrenogenital syndrome
    b) testicular feminization syndrome
    c) pure gonadal dysgenesis
    d) Turner's syndrome
240. Which of the following conditions show sex-chromatin positive cells?
    a) male pseudohermaphrodite
    b) testicular feminization syndrome
    c) Turner's syndrome
    d) Klinefelter's syndrome
241. The cremasteric fascia as a covering for the testis is derived from
    a) fascia transrversalis
    b) internal oblique muscle
    c) external oblique muscle
    d) processus vaginalis
242. When the processus vaginalis persists as a whole in the infant it leads to
    a) vaginal hydrocele
    b) infantile hydrocele
    c) congenital hydrocele
    d) hydrocele of cord
243. All of the following are the derivatives of the mesonephric duct in male **except**
    a) vas deferens
    b) ejaculatory duct
    c) appendix of epididymis
    d) appendix of testis
244. All of the following are the remnants of the mesonephric tubules **except**
    a) aberrant ductules of testis
    b) epididymis
    c) paraepididymis
    d) paroophoron
245. The cavity of mesencephalic vesicle of developing brain gives rise to
    a) lateral ventricle
    b) third ventricle
    c) fourth ventricle
    d) aqueduct of sylvius
246. All of the following are the derivatives of the neural crest **except**
    a) Schwann cells
    b) chromaffin cells
    c) adrenocortical cells
    d) melanoblasts
247. Which of the following is the derivative of the neural crest cells?
    a) pia mater
    b) astrocytes
    c) oligodendrocytes
    d) Schwann cells
248. Which of the following cells is derived from the mesoderm?
    a) microglia
    b) astrocytes
    c) oligodendrocytes
    d) Schwann cells

249. The dorsal nerve roots of spinal cord are formed by
   a) axons of the neurons located in dorsal horn of spinal cord
   b) axons of the neurons located in brain
   c) axons of the spinal ganglia cells
   d) all of the above

250. At full term the lower end of spinal cord lies at the level of which vertebral segment
   a) first lumbar
   b) third lumbar
   c) fifth lumbar
   d) second sacral

251. Optic vesicles are the outgrowths from
   a) telencephalon
   b) diencephalon
   c) mesencephalon
   d) rhombencephalon

252. Cerebellum is derived from
   a) myelencephalon
   b) metencephalon
   c) mesencephalon
   d) telencephalon

253. Intermediate horn of gray matter is developed in which region of the spinal cord?
   a) cervical
   b) thoracic and upper lumbar
   c) lower lumbar
   d) sacral

254. Which of the following cells loose their ability to divide once formed in the fetus
   a) hepatocytes
   b) lining epithelium of digestive tract
   c) neurons
   d) renal excretory cells

255. Which of the following nucleus contains the first order sensory neurons?
   a) main sensory nucleus of trigeminal nerve
   b) spinal nucleus of trigeminal nerve
   c) mesencephalic nucleus of trigeminal nerve
   d) nucleus solitarius

256. The enlargement of central canal of spinal cord is called as
   a) hydrocephalus
   b) hydromyelia
   c) meningomyelocele
   d) syringocele

GENETICS

257. Length of the mature human sperm is
    a) 20 to 60 micron
    b) 60 to 75 micron
    c) 200 to 600 micron
    d) 600 to 750 micron
258. Which of the following represent the facultative heterochromatin?
    a) diffuse, faintly staining nuclear chromatin
    b) clumped and densly staining chromatin all over the nucleus
    c) small pyknotic nucleus
    d) inactive X chromosome in female somatic cells
259. Which of the following is referred as the hereditary unit?
    a) chromosome
    b) gene
    c) nucleus
    d) RNA
260. 'Gene' can be defined as
    a) a segment of DNA responsible for production of a polypeptide or protein
    b) all the DNA on one chromosome
    c) all the DNA in the nucleus
    d) all the DNA and RNA of the nucleus
261. It was demonstrated that the human chromosome number is 46 only after the year
    a) 1856
    b) 1900
    c) 1956
    d) 1976
262. Which of the following defines the term centromere?
    a) end point of the chromosome
    b) each arm of the chromosome
    c) each strand in a double-stranded chromosome
    d) primary constriction where the chromatids are attached to each other
263. 'Acrocentric chromosome' is wherein the centromere is situated
    a) at the end.
    b) near the end.
    c) somewhere between the centre and the end of the chromosome.
    d) near the centre of chrosome.
264. Which of the following group of chromosomes shows satellites?
    a) Group A
    b) Group B
    c) Group C
    d) Group D

265. Apart from the nucleus which other cell organelle shows the presence of DNA?
    a) mitochondria
    b) ribosomes
    c) endoplasmic reticulum
    d) Golgi apparatus
266. Which of the following cell organelles are inherited to a child only from mother?
    a) mitochondria
    b) endoplasmic reticulum
    c) ribosomes
    d) Golgi apparatus
267. Which of the following statements concerning the euchromatic nucleus is/are correct?
    a) It is present in highly functional cells.
    b) In this the nucleus is stained evenly and faintly with nuclear dyes.
    c) It indicates that the genetic material is in the form of highly extended threads.
    d) All are correct.
268. Which of the following defines the nucleotide?
    a) single nitrogenous base bonded with the sugar
    b) single nitrogenous base bonded with single sugar-phosphate complex
    c) single nitrogenous base bonded with double sugar-phosphate complex
    d) two bases bonded together by hydrogen bonds
269. Which of the following phosphate moeity is present in the sugar-phosphate backbone of the polynucleotide?
    a) monophosphate
    b) diphosphate
    c) triphosphate
    d) any of the above
270. Which of the following is correct concerning the nitrogenous base pairing in the DNA molecule?
    a) $A \equiv T$
    b) $G = A$
    c) $C = A$
    d) $G \equiv C$
271. Which of the following statements concerning the mitochondrial DNA is correct?
    a) it does not encode for proteins
    b) it is inherited from both the parents equally
    c) it is in the form of rings
    d) all of the above are correct
272. Function/s of the glycoprotein molecule on the cell surface is
    a) cell adhesion
    b) contact inhibition
    c) cell-cell recognition
    d) all of the above
273. How much of the human genome is constituted by repetitive DNA?
    a) 10-30%
    b) 30-40%
    c) 40-60%
    d) 60-70%

Chapter III

Genetics

274. The genetic code (codon) consists of
   a) one base pair
   b) duplet of bases
   c) triplet of bases
   d) tetraplet of bases
275. The silent or nonfunctional units of the eukaryotic gene which are not transcribed in the mRNA are
   a) exons
   b) introns
   c) cistrons
   d) operon
276. Which of the following statements define genetic heterogenicity?
   a) The phenomena of a single gene responsible for a number of distinct and seemingly unrelated phenotypes.
   b) The phenomena whereby a single phenotype results from indepedent activity of several genes.
   c) When both members of an allelic pair are able to express themselves fully in the phenotype.
   d) All of the above.
277. Type of substitution in true genetic mutations involving single base when a purine base is substituted by a pyrimidine base is called as
   a) transcription
   b) translation
   c) transversion
   d) transition
278. The mechanism by which the intron-sequences are eliminated from the primary RNA transcript to form functional messenger RNA is
   a) capping
   b) polyadenylation
   c) mRNA splicing
   d) translation
279. Genes that move on and between chromosomes are called as
   a) overlapping genes
   b) jumping genes
   c) split genes
   d) structural genes
280. Which of the following indicates reverse genetics?
   a) DNA-protein-RNA
   b) DNA-RNA-protein
   c) protein-RNA-DNA
   d) all of the above
281. Number of different amino acids in human body are
   a) 4
   b) 10
   c) 20
   d) 64
282. How much of the human genome is occupied by the unique non-repetitive DNA?
   a) 30-40%
   b) 40-60%
   c) 60-70%
   d) 70-90%
283. Out of the four daughter molecules, how many DNA molecules will possess a strand from original DNA molecule in the second generation of DNA molecules after replication?
   a) 1
   b) 2
   c) 3
   d) all 4

284. Synthesis of RNA from the DNA template takes place in presence of the enzyme
    a) RNA polymerase
    b) DNA polymerase
    c) reverse transcriptase
    d) restriction endonuclease

285. Which of the following nitrogenous bases is **not** present in ribonucleic acid?
    a) adenine
    b) thymine
    c) cytocine
    d) guanine

286. Which of the following nitrogenous base is **not** present in the DNA molecule?
    a) adenine
    b) guanine
    c) uracil
    d) cytocine

287. Formation of polypeptide chain from the mature messenger RNA is known as
    a) replication
    b) transcription
    c) RNA-splicing
    d) translation

288. Which of the folloowing acts as an adapter during translation?
    a) mRNA
    b) tRNA
    c) rRNA
    d) amino acids

289. In which of the following conditions is seen a characteristic pedigree showing that first case in the family appears sporadically?
    a) autosomal recessive
    b) autosomal dominant
    c) X-linked dominant
    d) X-linked recessive

290. A raised frequency of consanguineous marriages is seen in the parents of patients suffering from which conditions?
    a) autosomal dominant
    b) autosomal recessive
    c) sex-linked dominant
    d) sex-linked recessive

291. In which of the following conditions only half of the sons of the heterozygous female will be affected?
    a) autosomal dominant
    b) autosomal recessive
    c) X-linked dominant
    d) X-linked recessive

292. In which of the following conditions, all of the daughter's would be carrier but none of the sons affected of an affected man?
    a) autosomal dominant
    b) autosomal recessive
    c) X-linked dominant
    d) X-linked recessive

293. All of the following are autosomal dominant conditions **except**
    a) neurofibromatosis
    b) achondroplaria
    c) hemophilia
    d) osteogenesis imperfecta

294. All of the following are autosomal recessive disorders **except**
    a) oculocutaneous albinism
    b) alkaptonuria
    c) sickle cell disease
    d) myotonic dystrophy

Chapter III

Genetics

295. All of the following are the X-linked recessive conditions **except**
    a) hemophilia
    b) colour blindness
    c) G-6-PD deficiency
    d) thalassemia
296. Which of the following is the X-linked dominant condition?
    a) vitamin D-resistant rickets
    b) thalassemia
    c) hemophilia
    d) achondroplasia
297. Which of the following RNA is soluble?
    a) m-RNA
    b) t-RNA
    c) r-RNA
    d) all of the above
298. A globular histone core around which a variable length of DNA molecule is wound is known as
    a) nucleosome
    b) nucleotide
    c) nucleoside
    d) solenoid
299. One or more alternative forms of a gene found at the same position on the homologous chromosomes is known as
    a) locus
    b) centromeres
    c) allele
    d) amorph
300. The mating of closely related individuals is known as
    a) random mating
    b) inbreeding
    c) positive assortative mating
    d) negative assortative mating
301. How many autosomes are present in a single haploid set of chromosomes?
    a) 23
    b) 22
    c) 44
    d) 46
302. When both members of an allelic pair are able to express themselves fully in the phenotype, the inheritance is called as
    a) codominant
    b) intermediate
    c) dominant
    d) recessive
303. When the trait is the result of a sharing of, or a partial expression of both alleles, the inheritance is called as
    a) codominant
    b) intermediate
    c) dominant
    d) recessive
304. 'ABO' blood group is the example of which inheritance?
    a) codominant
    b) intermediate
    c) dominant
    d) recessive
305. Which of the following is an example of intermediate inheritance?
    a) 'ABO' blood group
    b) sickle cell trait
    c) thalassemia
    d) all sex linked
306. Which of the following mendelian traits is often called as holandric?
    a) X-linked recessive
    b) X-linked dominant
    c) Y-linked
    d) all sex linked

307. Homozygous is an individual who at one particular locus on homologus chromosomes possesses
    a) two different alleles
    b) two identical alleles
    c) two different mutant alleles
    d) one mutant and one normal alleles
308. An allele which is expressed only when it is homozygous is called as
    a) dominant
    b) codominant
    c) recessive
    d) having intermediate inheritance
309. The incidence of autosomal dominant disorders in general population is
    a) 7%
    b) 4%
    c) 0.7%
    d) 2%
310. The mendelian trait characteristically seen only in sibs but not in parents of offsprings is
    a) autosomal dominant
    b) autosomal recessive
    c) X-linked dominant
    d) X-linked recessive
311. The trait transmitted by an affected heterozygote to half of his/her children on an average is
    a) autosomal dominant
    b) autsomal recessive
    c) X-linked dominant
    d) X-linked recessive
312. All of the following individuals will be affected **except**
    a) heterozygote for autosomal dominant trait
    b) homozygote for autosomal recessive trait
    c) heterozygote female for X-linked recessive trait
    d) hemizygous male for X-linked recessive trait
313. Ability of a gene to express phenotypically is known as
    a) expressivity
    b) penetrance
    c) pleiotropy
    d) heterogenicity
314. Trait which is never transmitted from father to son is
    a) autosomal dominant
    b) autosomal recessive
    c) X-linked
    d) Y-linked
315. Occurrence of two or more phenotypic characters in a given population in a frequency greater than would be expected on the basis of chance is known as
    a) linkage
    b) association
    c) pleiotropy
    d) genetic heterogenicity
316. Genes located on autosomes and expressed only in one sex as a trait are known as
    a) sex-linked
    b) sex-limited
    c) sex-controlled
    d) sex-influenced

Chapter III
Genetics 37

317. An individual containing cells derived from two different zygotes is
    a) mosaic
    b) hybrid
    c) chimera
    d) propositus

318. A functional grouping of DNA loci including several structural genes, an operator, a promotor and a regulator gene is called as
    a) codon
    b) exon
    c) intron
    d) operon

319. All of the following statements are correct regarding meiosis I of cell division **except**
    a) DNA replication occurs before it
    b) bivalents are formed by pairing of homologous chromosomes
    c) cross-over and interchange of chromatid segments takes place
    d) it results in two daughter cells each with 23 single-stranded chromosomes

320. Which of the following statments regarding second meiosis is correct?
    a) DNA synthesis occurs before it
    b) bivalents are formed by pairing of homologous chromosomes
    c) cross-over and interchange of chromatid segments takes place
    d) it results in two daughter cells each with 23 single stranded chromosomes

321. Primordial germ cells appear in
    a) wall of the amniotic cavity
    b) wall of the yolk sac
    c) extraembryonic mesoderm
    d) chorion

322. Single nitrogenous base bonded with hexose sugar is known as
    a) nucleotide
    b) polynucleotide
    c) nucleoside
    d) bi-nucleotide

323. Double stranded helix of polynucleotides with the associated proteins is known as a
    a) chromosome
    b) chromatid
    c) gene
    d) solenoid

324. The phenomena whereby a single phenotype results from independent activity of several genes is known as
    a) pleiotrophy
    b) codominant inheritance
    c) anticipation
    d) genetic heterogeneity

325. When both members of an allelic pair are able to express themselves fully in phenotype the inheritance is known as
    a) recessive
    b) dominant
    c) codominant
    d) mitochondrial

326. The phenomena by which certain genes function differently depending on whether they are maternally or patternally derived is known as
    a) anticipation
    b) pleiotrophy
    c) imprinting
    d) heterogeneity

327. The phenomena of a single gene responsible for a number of distinct and seemingly unrelated phenotypes is known as
   a) codominant inheritance
   b) anticipation
   c) pleiotrophy
   d) genetic heterogeneity

328. A phenomena associated with the fusion of male and female gamete nuclei is
   a) activation
   b) amphimixis
   c) spermiogenesis
   d) parthenogenesis

329. A phenomena by which a mature sperm forms an embryo without fertilization is known as
   a) spermiogenesis
   b) gametogenesis
   c) conception
   d) parthenogenesis

330. A phenomena which ensue upon the entry of spermatozoa in the ovum is known as
   a) parthenogenesis
   b) gametogenesis
   c) capacitation
   d) activation

331. A phenomena concerned with the transformation of a spermatid into a spermatozoa is
   a) activation
   b) parthenogenesis
   c) spermiogenesis
   d) spermatogenesis

332. In the female genital tract, removal of glycoprotein and seminal plasma proteins from the plasma membrane covering acrosomal region of sperm is known as
   a) acrosomal reaction
   b) capacitation
   c) spermiogenesis
   d) activation

333. Ability of the cell to form any type of body tissue is known as
   a) modulation
   b) totipotency
   c) differentiation
   d) capacitation

Chapter IV

GENERAL ANATOMY

334. 'Father of Anatomy' is
    a) Galen
    b) Herophilus
    c) Hippocrates
    d) Henry Gray
335. 'Father of Medicine' is
    a) Galen
    b) Herophilus
    c) Hippocrates
    d) Vesalius
336. Who is the 'Founder of Modern Anatomy'?
    a) Galen
    b) Herophilus
    c) Leonardo da Vinci
    d) Vasalius
337. 'Ontogeny' is the developmental history of a man
    a) since fertilization till death
    b) through evolution
    c) before birth
    d) after birth
338. 'Phylogeny' is the developmental history of a man
    a) through life
    b) through evolution
    c) before birth
    d) after birth
339. Which of the following is the position of the body in 'Anatomical position'?
    a) erect
    b) sitting
    c) lying down with face upwards
    d) lying down with face downwards
340. What is this position called as 'lying supine with buttocks at the edge of the table, the hips and knees fully flexed, and the feet fully strapped in position'
    a) supine
    b) prone
    c) lithotomy
    d) anatomical
341. Regarding the coronal plane, all of the following statements are correct **except**
    a) it is at right angle to the median plane
    b) it is at right angle to the sagital plane
    c) it is at right angle to the horizontal plane
    d) it divides the body into two equal halves
342. Plane at right angle to the long axis of a body segment is known as
    a) coronal plane
    b) sagittal plane
    c) horizontal plane
    d) transverse plane

343. The term 'rostral' means
    a) towards the tail
    b) towards the head
    c) towards the belly
    d) towards the back

344. 'Preaxial border' of upper limb is its
    a) anterior median line
    b) posterior median line
    c) outer border
    d) inner border

345. Which of the following is called as 'raphe'?
    a) fibrous, cord-like part of muscle
    b) a flat tendon
    c) band of interdigitating fibres of the tendons
    d) none of the above

346. Which of the following sentences describe 'abduction'?
    a) movement towards the central axis
    b) approximation of ventral surfaces
    c) approximation of dorsal surfaces
    d) movement away from the central axis

347. Position of midflexed forearm so that the palm faces downwards is described as its
    a) medial rotation
    b) lateral rotation
    c) pronation
    d) supination

348. The proportion of organic to inorganic matter in the bones is
    a) 1 : 3
    b) 1 : 2
    c) 1 : 1
    d) 2 : 3

349. Which of the following ligaments mainly consist of elastic tissue?
    a) ligamenta flava
    b) calcaneonavicular ligament
    c) sacro-iliac
    d) ileofemoral ligament

350. The precartilaginous model of bone arises from
    a) endoderm
    b) ectoderm
    c) mesoderm
    d) neuroectoderm

351. Extensive vascular channels are seen in the cartilage in
    a) adult life
    b) embryonic life
    c) late childhood
    d) none of the above

352. Bone grows in length at
    a) epiphysis
    b) metaphysis
    c) epiphyseal plate
    d) periosteum

353. The first bone to ossify in the body is
    a) clavicle
    b) femur
    c) vertebrae
    d) humerus

354. Ossification begins in intrauterine life during the
    a) second week
    b) third week
    c) fourth week
    d) fifth week

355. What percent of body calcium is stored in bones?
    a) 80%
    b) 90%
    c) 99%
    d) 100%
356. Which of the following ligaments is mainly composed of elastic tissue?
    a) apical ligament of dens
    b) anterior longitudinal ligament of vertebral column
    c) collateral ligaments of elbow joint
    d) interossicular ligament
357. Which of the following bursa around the knee joint communicates with the cavity of the joint?
    a) prepatellar
    b) suprapatellar
    c) superficial infrapatellar
    d) deep infrapatellar
358. Which of the following bursa usually communicates with the shoulder joint?
    a) subscapular
    b) subacromial
    c) supraspinatus
    d) all of the above
359. 'A portal system' can be defined as a system of vessels interposed between
    a) two arteries
    b) vein and artery
    c) two veins
    d) two capillary plexuses
360. Sinusoids are seen in all of the following organs **except**
    a) spleen
    b) liver
    c) pancreas
    d) parotid gland
361. Functional end arteries are terminal branches of arteries which
    a) do not anastomose
    b) show anastomosis with arteries but insufficient
    c) show extensive open anastomosis of adjucent arteries
    d) show anastomosis with a vein
362. What is mesotendon?
    a) middle part of the tendon
    b) part of tendon near the fleshy part of muscle
    c) the fold of synovial sheath which suspends it in the sheath
    d) site of attachment of tendon to bone
363. Lymphatic vessels are found in all of the following **except**
    a) gastrointenstinal tract
    b) liver
    c) testis
    d) eyeball
364. Which of the following body structures show the presence of lymphatic vessels?
    a) brain
    b) cartilage
    c) internal ear
    d) pancreas
365. Which of the following vessels show the presence of valves?
    a) lymphatics
    b) veins of the neck
    c) arteries
    d) capillaries

366. Which of the following is called as a resistance vessel?
    a) arteries
    b) arterioles
    c) capillaries
    d) sinusoids
367. Elastic artery is what type of vessel?
    a) reservior
    b) conducting
    c) resistance
    d) distribution
368. Endotheliocytes linning the inner surface of blood vessels are
    a) tall columnar
    b) low columnar
    c) cuboidal
    d) squamous
369. 'Fenestrated capillaries' are found in all of the following structures except
    a) pancreas
    b) renal glomeruli
    c) intenstinal villi
    d) brain
370. Which of the following structures shows presence of fenestrated capillaries?
    a) skin
    b) lung
    c) thyroid gland
    d) connective tissue
371. Which of the following structures exhibits an extreme example of sinusoids with discontinuous endothelium?
    a) spleen
    b) liver
    c) pancreas
    d) pituitary gland
372. In larger veins which of the tunics is thickest?
    a) tunica intima
    b) tunica media
    c) tunica adventitia
    d) all tunics are of equal thickness
373. Non-striated myocytes appear throughout the adventitia in all of the following veins except
    a) inferior vena cava
    b) portal vein
    c) renal vein
    d) external iliac veins
374. Nonstriated muscle fibres are seen in the wall of
    a) decidual veins of placenta
    b) veins of trabecular bone
    c) retinal veins
    d) azygous vein
375. 'Countercurrent exchange' of heat between closely apposed arteries and veins is seen in
    a) renal medulla
    b) hypophysis cerebri
    c) intenstinal villi
    d) testis
376. Bleeding occurs from both the cut ends when the sectioned vessel is
    a) artery
    b) vein
    c) arteriovenous anastomotic channel
    d) interarterial anastomotic channel

377. Specialized arteriovenous anastomoses are seen in
    a) the skin of the hands
    b) alimentary mucosa
    c) tongue
    d) thyroid gland
378. All of the following are non-striated muscles **except**
    a) arrector pilorum
    b) dartos muscle of scrotum
    c) palmaris brevis
    d) muscles of iris
379. All of the following sites show admixture of smooth and striated muscle **except**
    a) anal shincter
    b) soft palate
    c) upper eyelid
    d) intermediate zone of oesophagus
380. Myocyte containing numerous nuclei is/are
    a) cardiac
    b) smooth
    c) skeletal
    d) all of the above
381. In the skeletal muscle fibre, nuclei are especially numerus in the **region** of
    a) muscle origin
    b) muscle insertion
    c) middle of fibre
    d) neuromuscular junction
382. Connective tissue sheath enclosing the individual muscle fibre in the skeletal muscle is called as
    a) sarcolemma
    b) epimycium
    c) perimycium
    d) endomycium
383. When skeletal muscle fibre contracts the contraction band appears on either side of which band?
    a) A
    b) I
    c) Z
    d) H
384. In a relaxed muscle, the region of sarcomere where actin filaments are absent is represented by
    a) A band
    b) I band
    c) H band
    d) Z band
385. In the skeletal muscle fibre the thickness of actin filament is
    a) 3 nm
    b) 6 nm
    c) 9 nm
    d) 12 nm
386. 'Sarcomere' is the portion of myofilament between which of the two adjucant bands
    a) A
    b) Z
    c) H
    d) M
387. Motor nerve fibres to the muscle spindles are
    a) alpha efferents
    b) gamma efferents
    c) autonomic efferents
    d) all of the above

388. A 'motor unit' is defined as the combination of
   a) an alpha motor neuron with all the muscle fibres which it innervates
   b) a gamma neuron with all the muscle spindles which it innervates
   c) a nerve with all the muscles it innervates
   d) a spinal segment with all the muscles it supplies

389. All of the following are characteristics of cardiac muscle **except**
   a) intercalated disc
   b) striations
   c) involuntary
   d) multinucleated

390. Spontaneous rhythmic contractions occur in the following structure **except**
   a) stomach
   b) vas deference
   c) uterus
   d) ureter

391. All of the following structures have scarce blood supply **except**
   a) tendons
   b) bones
   c) cartilages
   d) ligaments

392. Superficial fascia is absent in
   a) scalp
   b) palm
   c) sole
   d) ear pinna

393. Pull of the following muscles is transmitted to the bone through the deep fascia **except**
   a) palmaris brevis
   b) biceps femoris
   c) biceps brachii
   d) gluteus maximus

394. Which of the following muscles in human body has longest muscle fibres?
   a) deltoid
   b) gluteus maximus
   c) gastrocnemius
   d) sartorius

395. Tendinous intersections are seen in which of the following muscles?
   a) rectus femoris
   b) rectus abdominis
   c) gluteus maximus
   d) lattissimus dorsi

396. Which of the following is a circumpennate muscle?
   a) deltoid
   b) rectus femoris
   c) tibialis anterior
   d) rectus abdominis

397. Which of the following is the unipennate muscle?
   a) rectus femoris
   b) dorsal interossei
   c) flexor pollicis longus
   d) deltoid

398. What type of muscle the deltoid is?
   a) unipennate
   b) bipennate
   c) circumpennate
   d) multipennate

399. In following muscles, muscle fibres are spirally arranged **except**
   a) rectus abdominis
   b) trapezius
   c) sternocleidomastoid
   d) lattissimus dorsi

Chapter IV General Anatomy 45

400. In flexion of elbow, triceps acts as a
   a) prime mover
   b) fixator
   c) synergist
   d) antagonist
401. Muscles eliminating unwanted movements produced by prime movers are called as
   a) antagonists
   b) synergists
   c) fixators
   d) prime movers
402. 'Head' is the part of all of the following bones **except**
   a) radius
   b) tibia
   c) humerus
   d) femur
403. Costovertebral joint is of which type?
   a) hinge
   b) ellipsoid
   c) plane
   d) synchondrosis
404. The lower facet on the head of a typical rib articulates with the demifacet on
   a) inferior part of corresponding vertebra
   b) superior part of corresponding vertebra
   c) superior part of vertebra below the corresponding vertebra
   d) inferior part of vetebra below the corresponding vetebra
405. All of the following ribs articulate only with one vertebra **except**
   a) first
   b) ninth
   c) twelfth
   d) eleventh
406. The tubercle of a typical rib articulates with the facet on the transverse process of
   a) its own vertebra
   b) vertebra above
   c) vertebra below
   d) all of the above
407. Aperture through which spinal nerve passes is bounded by the vertebral body and
   a) lateral costotransverse ligament
   b) superior costotransverse ligament
   c) intraarticular ligament
   d) none of the above
408. Which of the following ribs articulates with the transverse process of vertebra?
   a) first
   b) eleventh
   c) twelfth
   d) none of the above
409. Which of the following ribs do not articulate with the transverse process of vertebra?
   a) first
   b) second
   c) tenth
   d) eleventh
410. In sternocostal joints of 2nd to 7th costal cartilages, the joint **cavities** are
   a) often absent in upper joints
   b) often absent in lower joints
   c) absent in all joints
   d) present in all joints

411. All of the following statements regarding manubriosternal joints are true **except**
    a) it is a symphysis type of joint
    b) in about 30% of people it shows synovial joint cavity
    c) it moves slightly during respiration
    d) the sternal angle indicates manubriosternal joint
412. Which of the following is a primary cartilageous joint?
    a) manubriosternal
    b) xiphisternal
    c) intervertebral
    d) costovertebral
413. Transverse diameter of thorax increases by
    a) bucket-handle movement of ribs
    b) pump handle movement of ribs
    c) diaphragmatic contraction
    d) diaphragmatic relaxation
414. Anteroposterior diameter of thorax increases by
    a) bucket-handle movement of ribs
    b) pump handle movement of ribs
    c) diaphragmatic contraction
    d) diaphragmatic relaxation
415. Vertical diameter of thorax increases by
    a) bucket-handle movement of ribs
    b) pump handle movement of ribs
    c) diaphragmatic contraction
    d) diaphragmatic relaxation
416. Strongest ligament in the body is
    a) ileofemoral
    b) cruciate ligaments
    c) lateral collateral ligament of elbow
    d) interosseous sacroiliac
417. What type of joint sacroiliac is?
    a) primary cartilaginous
    b) secondary cartilaginous
    c) plane synovial
    d) ellipsoid
418. Sacroiliac joints differ from most synovial joints in the body because
    a) they do not have synovial cavity
    b) they do not have capsule
    c) they possess very little mobility
    d) there is no articular cartilage covering the bony surfaces
419. The sacroiliac joints are softer and more yielding in
    a) children
    b) old age
    c) late pregnancy in women
    d) through out life
420. Artery to the head of femur is a branch of
    a) anterior division of obturator artery
    b) posterior division of obturator artery
    c) superficial circumflex iliac artery
    d) lateral circumflex artery

421. All of the following nerves innervate hip joint **except**
    a) femoral
    b) obturator
    c) inferior gluteal
    d) sciatic
422. In syndesmosis, which of the following structures connects the two bones?
    a) collagenous sutural ligament
    b) collagenous interosseous ligament
    c) hyaline cartilage
    d) fibrocartilage
423. All of the following are sutural type of joints **except**
    a) serrate
    b) schindylesis
    c) sellar
    d) limbous
424. Which of the following joints is a gomphosis?
    a) dentatoalveolar
    b) manubriosternal
    c) denticulate suture
    d) interosseous radioulnar
425. All of the following joints are symphyses **except**
    a) acromioclavicular
    b) intervertebral
    c) pubic symphysis
    d) manubriosternal
426. Synostosis can be defined as union of bones by
    a) interosseous ligaments
    b) hyline cartilage
    c) fibrocartilage
    d) bone
427. What type of joint is present between the epiphysis and diaphysis of long bones?
    a) primary cartilaginous
    b) secondary cartilaginous
    c) synovial
    d) fibrous
428. All of the following characteristics regarding articular cartilage surface are true **except**
    a) wear resistant
    b) high frictional
    c) lubrication
    d) slightly compressible
429. Articular cartilages having convex surfaces are
    a) thickest centrally, thinning peripherally
    b) thickest peripherally and thinning centrally
    c) even in thickness throughout
    d) of irregular thickness
430. Which of the following is **not** a source of nourishment of articular cartilage?
    a) direct arterial supply
    b) synovial fluid
    c) vascular plexus in synovial membrane
    d) blood vessels in adjacent marrow spaces.

431. Which of the following statements regarding articular cartilage is correct?
    a) It is highly vascular.
    b) It is devoid of perichondrium.
    c) It is covered by synovial membrane.
    d) It has no nerves.
432. All of the following statements regarding ligaments of the joints are true **except**
    a) **intrinsic** ligaments are local thickenings of the capsule.
    b) accessory ligaments are separate from capsule.
    c) accessory ligaments are always extracapsular.
    d) ligaments do not resist normal actions.
433. All of the following intraarticular structures are lined by synovial membrane **except**
    a) non-articulating bone surface
    b) menisci
    c) ligaments
    d) tendons
434. All of the following statements regarding primary cartilaginous joints are correct **except**
    a) bones are united by hyaline cartilage
    b) slight bending is permitted at these joints
    c) growth in length of bone is permitted at these joints
    d) this type of joint is a permanent joint
435. Symphyses are also called as
    a) fibrocartilaginous joints
    b) synchondroses
    c) primary cartilaginous joints
    d) syndesmoses
436. First sternochondral joint is
    a) a permanant synchondrosis
    b) a temporary synchondrosis
    c) fibrocartilaginous joint
    d) syndesmosis
437. Symphysis menti is
    a) a primary cartilaginous joint
    b) a secondary cartilaginous joint
    c) a synovial joint
    d) a syndesmosis
438. All of the following are the distinguishing features of a synovial joint **except**
    a) a joint cavity
    b) an articular cartilage
    c) an articular capsule
    d) epiphyseal cartilaginous plate
439. Articular surfaces of bones in synovial joints are covered by
    a) synovial membrane
    b) articular cartilage
    c) joint capsule
    d) periosteum
440. Synovial membrane in synovial joints **does not cover**
    a) inner surface of joint capsule
    b) articular cartilage
    c) **intracapsular parts of bone**
    d) intracapsular ligaments

Chapter IV

General Anatomy

441. All of the following statements regarding synovial membrane are correct **except**
     a) it is a part of the fibrous capsule
     b) it is avascular
     c) it regenerates if damaged
     d) it produces lubricating fluid
442. Which of the following joints shows the presence of an articular disc?
     a) ankle joint
     b) elbow joint
     c) wrist joint
     d) first carpometacarpal joint
443. Which of the following joints **does not show** the presence of articular disc?
     a) temporomandibular
     b) wrist
     c) sternoclavicular
     d) elbow
444. Fibrocartilaginous labrum is present in
     a) shoulder joint
     b) knee joint
     c) temporomandibular joint
     d) all of the above
445. All of the following statements regarding hinge joint are correct **except**
     a) they move only in one axis
     b) they permit extension and flexion only
     c) bones are joined by strong collateral ligaments
     d) the articular capsule of these joints is very thick
446. Condyloid joints are
     a) uniaxial
     b) biaxial
     c) polyaxial
     d) immobile
447. Which of the following is a hinge joint?
     a) elbow
     b) wrist
     c) superior radioulnar
     d) talocalcaneonavicular
448. Which of the following is a saddle joint?
     a) knee
     b) wrist
     c) first carpometacarpal
     d) elbow
449. All of the following are ball and socket type of joints **except**
     a) talocalcaneonavicular
     b) shoulder
     c) hip
     d) temporomandibular
450. Which of the following is **not** a pivot joint?
     a) superior radioulnar
     b) inferior radioulnar
     c) first carpometacarpal
     d) middle atalantoaxial
451. 'Hilton's law' states that
     a) the nerve of the joints also supplies the muscles and the skin over it
     b) muscle covering the joints act on the joint
     c) artery of the joint also supplies the muscles and the skin over it
     d) pain fibres are numerous in the fibrous capsule

452. Regarding joint pain all of the following statements are correct **except**
   a) excessive streching of the joint capsule is very painful
   b) synovial membrane is higly sensitive
   c) joint pain is poorly localized
   d) injury to one joint can cause referred pain in another joint

453. Menisci are found in which of the following joint?
   a) stenoclavicular
   b) shoulder
   c) temporomandibular
   d) knee

454. All of the following joints show presence of a complete fibrocartilaginous disc **except**
   a) sternoclavicular
   b) shoulder
   c) inferior radioulnar
   d) temporomandibular

455. All of the following structures are intra-articular **except**
   a) bursa
   b) labrum
   c) fat pads
   d) menisci

456. Which of the following is called as a labrum?
   a) fibrocartilaginous annular lip
   b) complete fibrocartilaginous disc
   c) incomplete fibrocartilaginous disc
   d) articular hyaline cartilage

457. The thickness of articular cartilages in youth in larger joints may reach upto
   a) 1-2 mm
   b) 0.1-0.2 mm
   c) 0.5-0.7 mm
   d) 5-7 mm

458. Once the synoviocyte ingests the particulate matter it
   a) migrates to the synovial cavity
   b) migrates to the subintimal layer
   c) remains in intimal layer
   d) degenerates

459. In human joints the synovial fluid in synovial joints is not more than
   a) 0.05 ml
   b) 0.5 ml
   c) 5 ml
   d) 10 ml

460. Translation of joint is
   a) simple sliding movement
   b) sliding with appreciable angulation
   c) sliding with appreciable rotation
   d) none of the above

461. Which of the following joints does not exhibit flexion-extension in the sagittal plane?
   a) shoulder
   b) elbow
   c) hip
   d) knee

Chapter IV

General Anatomy 51

462. Which of the following joints does not exhibit adduction-abduction around its anteroposterior axis?
    a) pollicial carpometacarpal
    b) hip
    c) wrist
    d) carpometacarpal other than pollicial

463. Movement of humerus in the scapular plane around an axis at right angle to it is
    a) adduction
    b) abduction
    c) flexion
    d) extension

464. Adjunct rotation is
    a) indepedent rotation
    b) combined with some other movement
    c) combined with translation
    d) all of the above

465. When any bone is solely rotating around its stationary mechanical axis, it is said to show
    a) pure swing
    b) pure spin
    c) impure swing
    d) impure spin

466. All of the following statements about the fully close-packed joint are correct **except**
    a) articular surfaces are fully cogruant
    b) articular surfaces are in maximal contact
    c) articular surfaces are tightly compressed
    d) fibrous capsule and ligaments are maximally relaxed

467. Temporomandibular joint is
    a) condylar
    b) saddle
    c) hinge
    d) pivot

468. Lateral temporomandibular ligament is attached above to
    a) the squamotympanic fissure
    b) mandibular fossa
    c) articular tubercle
    d) all of the above

469. All of the following structures separate the sphenomandibular ligament from the mandible **except**
    a) maxillary vessels
    b) inferior alveolar vessels
    c) maxillary nerve
    d) inferior alveolar nerve

470. Which of the following parts of mandible gives attachment to sphenomandibular ligament?
    a) neck a mandible
    b) coronoid process
    c) angle fo mandible
    d) lingula of mandibular foramen

471. Which of the following nerves pierces the sphenomandibular ligament?
    a) nerve to mylohyoid
    b) inferior alveolar nerve
    c) lingual nerve
    d) chorda tympani nerve

472. Which of the following structures is related to the sphenomandibular ligament medially?
   a) chorda tympani nerve
   b) inferior alveolar nerve
   c) maxillary vessels
   d) parotid lobule

473. Temporomandibular joint is innervated by which of the following nerves?
   a) auriculotemporal
   b) inferior alveolar
   c) lingual
   d) maxillary

474. Which of the following muscles is **not** a depressor of mandible?
   a) lateral pterygoid
   b) medial pterygoid
   c) diagastric
   d) geniohyoid

475. Which of the following muscles is the retractor of the mandible?
   a) lateral pterygoid
   b) medial pterygoid
   c) temporalis
   d) mylohyoid

476. Which of the following mandibular movements is not performed by lateral pterygoid?
   a) depression
   b) protrusion
   c) retraction
   d) side to side movements

477. With the mouth open, a sudden violence may dislocate the mandibular head
   a) only forwards
   b) only backwards
   c) only laterally
   d) in any direction

478. Reduction of dislocated mandible involves
   a) depressing the chin and elevating the jaw posteriorly
   b) depressing the jaw posteriorly and elevating the chin
   c) depressing the jaw and depressing the chin
   d) elevating the jaw posteriosly and elevating the chin

479. Which of the following ligaments is continuous above as membrana tectoria?
   a) anterior longitudinal
   b) posterior longitudinal
   c) ligamenta flava
   d) ligamentum nuchae

480. Between which of the following vertebrae, intervertebral disc is absent?
   a) first and second cervical vertebra
   b) last cervical and first thoracic vertebra
   c) last thoracic and first lumbar vertebra
   d) last lumbar vertebra and sacrum

481. Which of the following statements regarding the intervertebral discs is correct?
   a) it has reached blood supply
   b) it is totally avascular
   c) its peripheral part only is vascular
   d) its central part only is vascular

482. In old age strain on the intevertebral disc may cause bulge of annulus pulposus
    a) anteromedially
    b) anterolaterally
    c) posteromedially
    d) posterolaterally

483. Which of the following ligaments is formed mainly by elastic tissue?
    a) anterior longitudinal
    b) posterior longitudinal
    c) ligamenta flava
    d) ligamentum nuchae

484. Between the seventh cervical spine and external occipital protruberance which of the following ligaments is expanded as ligamentum nuchae?
    a) ligamenta flava
    b) posterior longitudinal
    c) interspinous
    d) supraspinous

485. Superior and inferior vertebral notches are almost of equal depth in intervertebral foramina of
    a) cervical region
    b) thoracic region
    c) lumbar region
    d) all of the above

486. All of the following are contents of intervertebral foramina **except**
    a) vertebral arteries
    b) segmental spinal nerves
    c) recurrent meningeal nerves
    d) spinal arteries

487. In the vertebral column flexion is most extensive at
    a) cervical level
    b) thoracic level
    c) lumbar level
    d) sacral level

488. Articulation of atlas to axis is at how many synovial joints?
    a) one
    b) two
    c) three
    d) four

489. The median atlantoaxial joint is
    a) pivot
    b) hinge
    c) condylar
    d) plane

490. The lateral atlantoaxial joint is
    a) pivot
    b) hinge
    c) condylar
    d) plane

491. The median atlantoaxial joint has how many synovial cavities?
    a) one
    b) two
    c) three
    d) four

492. Anterior articular surface of transverse ligament of atlantoaxial joint is
    a) fibrous
    b) bony
    c) cartilaginous
    d) osseo-cartilaginous

493. The upper band of atlantal cruciform ligament lies
    a) between basiocciput and apical ligament
    b) between apical ligament and membrana tectoria
    c) behind membrana tectoria
    d) between dens and medial tubercle of lateral mass of atlas

494. Movement at atlantoaxial joint involves
    a) rotation of dens in the ring of atlas
    b) rotation of atlas on the axis
    c) rotation of both atlas and axis in reverse direction
    d) no rotation

495. Atlantal facets for atlantooccipital joints are
    a) concave and centrally not constricted
    b) concave and centrally constricted
    c) convex and not constricted
    d) convex and constricted

496. Which of the following membranes arches over the groove for the vertebral artery on the arch of atlas?
    a) anterior atlantooccipital membrane
    b) membrana tectoria
    c) posterior atlantooccipital membrane
    d) none of the above

497. Which of the following movements is possible at atlantooccipital joint?
    a) adduction-abduction
    b) rotation
    c) flexion-extension
    d) circumduction

498. Alar ligaments connecting dens of axis with occipital bone
    a) relax in extension
    b) tauten in extension
    c) relax in flexion
    d) remain taut all the time

499. All of the following statements regarding apical ligament of dens are true **except**
    a) it extends from apex of dens to margin of foramen magnum
    b) it lies between alar ligaments
    c) it blends with deep fibres of posterior atlantooccipital membrane
    d) it is said to contain traces of notocord.

500. All of the following cells of general connective tissue, represent a fluctuating population of immigrant, wandering cells **except**
    a) macrophages
    b) fibroblasts
    c) mast cells
    d) lymphocytes

501. Which of the following cells of general connective tissue serve as a defensive cell in body?
    a) macrophages
    b) fibroblasts
    c) adipocytes
    d) mesenchymal stem cells

502. Which of the following tissues is predominantly composed of intercellular material, secreted by its own cells which are widely spaced?
    a) epithelial tissue
    b) connective tissue
    c) muscular tissue
    d) nervous tissue

503. Which of the following structures contain regular connective tissue?
    a) reticular layer of dermis
    b) sclera of the eye
    c) ligaments
    d) periosteum

Chapter IV

504. 'Panniculus adiposus' is the term used to refer the abundant adipose tissue.
    a) around the kidneys
    b) behind the eyeball
    c) in the subcutaneous tissue
    d) in the female breasts
505. Which of the following types of cartilages is not seen in human being?
    a) hyaline
    b) cellular
    c) yellow elastic
    d) white fibrocartilage
506. Which of the following is an example of elastic cartilage?
    a) costal
    b) nasal
    c) articular discs
    d) epiglottis
507. All the following terms describe the sternoclavicular joint **except**
    a) synovial
    b) complex
    c) ellipsoid
    d) compound
508. When bones are joined by hyaline cartilage, the resultant joint is
    a) symphysis
    b) synchondrosis
    c) synostosis
    d) syndesmosis

Chapter V

UPPER LIMB

509. Which of the following structures shows suprasternal ossicles when present?
   a) the interclavicular ligament
   b) anterior sternoclavicular ligament
   c) costoclavicular ligament
   d) articular disc of sternoclavicular joint

510. Sternoclavicular and acromioclavicular joints together permit the scapular rotation of about
   a) 30°
   b) 60°
   c) 90°
   d) 120°

511. Close-packing of acromioclavicular joint occurs when the angle between the superior scapular border and clavicular shaft reaches about
   a) 30°
   b) 60°
   c) 90°
   d) 120°

512. Which of the following statements is true concerning acromioclavicular dislocation?
   a) coracoclavicular ligament remains intact
   b) scapula falls away from the clavicle
   c) it never occurs
   d) it is always associated with fracture clavicle

513. Protraction of scapula is not involved in
   a) shoulder shrugging
   b) pushing
   c) thrusting
   d) reaching movements

514. Forward rotation of scapula is always associated with
   a) humeral rotation
   b) protraction of scapula
   c) retraction of scapula
   d) depression of lateral end of clavicle

515. Which of the following is not involved in coracoacromial arch formation?
   a) coracoclavicular ligament
   b) coracoid process
   c) acromion process
   d) coracoacromial ligament

516. Close-packing position of the shoulder joint is reached when the humerus is
   a) adducted and laterally rotated
   b) adducted and medially rotated
   c) abducted and medially rotated
   d) abducted and laterally rotated

Chapter V   Upper Limb   57

517. Attachment of fibrous capsule of shoulder joint on humerus descends more than one centimeter on the humeral shaft
    a) anterolaterally
    b) posterolaterally
    c) inferomedially
    d) inferolaterally
518. All of the following muscles form the rotator cuff for shoulder joint **except**
    a) supraspinatus
    b) subscapularis
    c) teres minor
    d) long head of triceps
519. Long head of triceps is separated from capsule of shoulder joint by
    a) radial nerve
    b) axillary nerve
    c) median nerve
    d) ulnar nerve
520. Which of the following structures acts as a retinaculum for the tendon of long head of biceps brachi?
    a) coracohumeral ligament
    b) transverse humeral ligament
    c) glenohumeral ligaments
    d) glenoidal labrum
521. All of the following nerves supply the shoulder joint **except**
    a) axillary
    b) lateral pectoral
    c) suprascapular
    d) musculocutaneous
522. With the arm dependent, when moderately loaded, downward displacement of humerus is prevented by
    a) pectoralis major
    b) infraspinatus
    c) supraspinatus
    d) subscapularis
523. Pure abduction at shoulder joint raises the arm
    a) anterolaterally
    b) laterally in coronal plane
    c) posterolaterally
    d) medially
524. In pure flexion-extension of arm the axis of movement is
    a) parallel to the glenoid cavity
    b) the long axis of humerus
    c) projected from the centre of the glenoid cavity
    d) anteroposterior axis through shoulder joint
525. Which of the following muscles is responsible for medial rotation of humerus?
    a) supraspinatus
    b) infraspinatus
    c) teres minor
    d) lattissimus dorsi
526. All of the following muscles are responsible for flexion of arm **except**
    a) pectoralis major
    b) pectoralis minor
    c) anterior fibres of deltoid
    d) coracobrachialis
527. When shoulder joint ankyloses, to make full use of the scapular mobility, the arm should be
    a) abducted
    b) adducted
    c) flexed
    d) extended

528. All of the following parts in elbow joint are covered by synovial membrane **except**
    a) medial trochlear surface
    b) capitulum
    c) lower part of annular ligament
    d) olecranon fossa

529. Which of the following branches of musculocutaneous nerve supply the elbow joint?
    a) coracobrachialis
    b) biceps brachii
    c) brachialis
    d) lateral cutaneous nerve of forearm

530. Carrying angle is about
    a) 20 degree
    b) 120 degree
    c) 160 degree
    d) 180 degree

531. Carrying angle is measured in
    a) full extension of forearm in supination
    b) midflexion of forearm
    c) pronation of extended forearm
    d) full flexion of forearm

532. Which of the following muscles acts at elbow most effectively in midprone position?
    a) pronator teres
    b) extensor carpi radialis
    c) brachioradialis
    d) flexor carpi radialis

533. All of the following statements regarding clavicle are correct **except**
    a) it is the only horizontally placed bone in the body
    b) it has no medullary cavity
    c) it develops from two primary centres of ossification
    d) it is subcutaneous throughout

534. Developmentally, which of the following long bones is a membrano-cartilaginous one?
    a) femur
    b) humerus
    c) clavicle
    d) fibula

535. The only long bone in the body with two primary centres of ossification is
    a) femur
    b) clavicle
    c) humerus
    d) radius

536. The earliest bone to ossify in the body is
    a) femur
    b) scapula
    c) clavicle
    d) tibia

537. Nutrient artery to the humerus is a branch of which artery?
    a) brachial
    b) profunda branchii
    c) anterior circumflex humeral
    d) superior ulnar collateral

538. The most common site of fracture of the clavicle is the junction between
    a) medial and lateral half
    b) middle and lateral thirds
    c) middle and medial thirds
    d) lateral 3/4 and medial 1/4
539. Structure passing through the suprascapular foramen is
    a) suprascapular artery
    b) suprascapular vein
    c) suprascapular nerve
    d) supraspinatus muscle
540. Glenoid cavity of the scapula is directed
    a) upwards, forwards and laterally
    b) upwards, backwards and laterally
    c) downwards, forwards and laterally
    d) downwards, backwards and laterally
541. The coracoid process of scapula represents
    a) traction epiphysis
    b) pressure epiphysis
    c) atavastic epiphysis
    d) none of the above
542. Following arteries take part in anastomosis around scapula **except**
    a) suprascapular
    b) dorsal scapular
    c) circumflex scapular
    d) thoracoacromial
543. Winging of scapula occurs due to damage to
    a) suprascapular nerve
    b) upper subscapular nerve
    c) long thoracic nerve
    d) dorsal scapular nerve
544. Which of the thoracic spines correspond with the inferior angle of scaula?
    a) fifth
    b) seventh
    c) ninth
    d) twelfth
545. Following muscles connect the scapula to the vertebral column **except**
    a) subscapularis
    b) levator scapulae
    c) trapezius
    d) lattissimus dorsi
546. "Deltoid tubercle" is the term erroneously used for
    a) site of insertion of deltoid muscle
    b) site of origin of deltoid muscle
    c) attachment of trapezius on the root of scapular spine
    d) muscle belly of deltoid muscle
547. Anatomical neck of humerus is
    a) margin of articular head of humerus
    b) line where upper end tapers to become continuous with shaft
    c) line joining lower ends of greater and lesser tubercles of humerus
    d) margin of articular surface of lower end of humerus
548. Intertubercular sulcus of humerus contains
    a) long head of biceps brachii
    b) branch of anterior circumflex humeral artery
    c) insertion of lattissimus dorsi
    d) all of the above

549. Head of humerus is directed
    a) upwards, backwards and medially
    b) downwards, backwards and medially
    c) upwards, forwards and medially
    d) upwards, backwards, laterally
550. Nerve most likely to be damaged in fracture of surgical neck of humerus is
    a) radial
    b) ulnar
    c) axillary
    d) musculocutaneous
551. Nerve most likely to be damaged in fracture of shaft of humerus is
    a) radial
    b) axillary
    c) ulnar
    d) median
552. Condylar fracture of humerus may cause damage to which of the following nerves?
    a) radial
    b) ulnar
    c) median
    d) axillary
553. All of the following nerves are intimately related to humerus **except**
    a) median
    b) radial
    c) ulnar
    d) axillary
554. 'Surgical neck' of humerus is in direct relation to all of the following structures **except**
    a) axillary artery
    b) axillary nerve
    c) anterior circumflex humeral artery
    d) posterior circumflex humeral artery
555. Spiral groove of humerus contains
    a) axillary nerve
    b) brachial artery
    c) radial nerve
    d) ulnar nerve
556. Following muscles are the superficial extensors of forearm **except**
    a) extensor pollicis longus
    b) extensor carpi radialis
    c) extensor carpi ulnaris
    d) extensor digiti minimi
557. Nerve lodged in the groove behind medial epicondyle of humerus is
    a) radial
    b) median
    c) musculocutaneous
    d) ulnar
558. 'Angle of humeral torsion' is the angle between the
    a) longest axes of proximal and distal articular surfaces
    b) long axis of upper end and long axis of shaft
    c) long axis of shaft and that of lower end
    d) none of the above
559. Elbow joint is what type of joint?
    a) pivot
    b) saddle
    c) ball and socket
    d) hinge

Chapter V   Upper Limb   61

560. Superior radioulnar joint is what type of joint?
    a) pivot   b) saddle
    c) hinge   d) plane
561. All of the following are pivot joints **except**
    a) atlantoccipital   b) superior radioulnar
    c) inferior radioulnar   d) atlantoaxial median
562. Oblique cord of forearm is the fibrous remnant of embryological head of
    a) flexor pollicis longus   b) flexor digitorum superficialis
    c) flexor digitorum profundus   d) pronator teres
563. The groove on the medial side of dorsal tubercle of radius transmits tendon of
    a) extensor carpi radialis   b) extensor pollicis longus
    c) extensor digitorum longus   d) extensor digiti minimi
564. Carpal bone which fractures most freuqentely is
    a) scaphoid   b) lunate
    c) hamate   d) capitate
565. First carpometacarpal joint is
    a) saddle   b) ellipsoid
    c) hinge   d) pivot
566. Which of the following joints contains the labrum?
    a) shoulder   b) wrist
    c) elbow   d) first metacarpophalangeal
567. Articular surface of sternal end of clavicle is covered by
    a) fibrocartilage   b) elastic cartilage
    c) hyaline cartilage   d) none of the above
568. Which of the following joints contains articular disc?
    a) sternoclavicular   b) elbow
    c) superior radioulnar   d) shoulder
569. Which of the following muscles causes protraction of scapula?
    a) trapezius   b) levator scapulae
    c) serratus anterior   d) lattissimus dorsi
570. Which of the following muscles is reponsible for initial 15 degree abduction at shoulder joint?
    a) subscapularis   b) deltoid
    c) supraspinatus   d) infraspinatus
571. All of the following are the lateral rotators of arm **except**
    a) teres major   b) infraspinatus
    c) teres minor   d) posterior fibres of deltoid
572. Which of the following muscles is supplied by double nerves?
    a) pronator teres   b) flexor digitorum superficialis
    c) flexor pollicis longus   d) flexor digitorum profundus

573. Trapezius retracts the scapula along with which of the following muscles?
    a) levator scapulae
    b) rhombodeus
    c) serratus anterior
    d) lattissimus dorsi

574. Which of the following muscles of upper limb is supplied by a cranial nerve?
    a) levator scapulae
    b) deltoid
    c) pectoralis major
    d) trapezius

575. Lattissimus dorsi is supplied by
    a) long thoracic nerve
    b) thoracodorsal nerve
    c) suprascapular nerve
    d) subscapular nerve

576. Which of the following muscles acts as adductor, extensor and medial rotator of arm?
    a) pectoralis major
    b) teres minor
    c) infraspinatus
    d) lattissimus dorsi

577. All of the following are medial rotators of arm **except**
    a) subscapularis
    b) teres major
    c) lattissimus dorsi
    d) coracobrachialis

578. All of the following form the boundaries of 'lumbar triangle' **except**
    a) quadratus lumborum
    b) iliac crest
    c) external oblique abdominis
    d) lattissimus dorsi

579. Triangle of auscultation is bounded by all of the following muscles **except**
    a) lattissimus dorsi
    b) medial border of scapula
    c) trapezius
    d) quadratus lumborum

580. Which of the following muscles join shoulder and the pelvic girdle together?
    a) trapezius
    b) quadratus lumborum
    c) external oblique abdominis
    d) lattissimus dorsi

581. Axillary nerve supplies which of the following muscles?
    a) supraspinatus
    b) teres major
    c) teres minor
    d) infraspinatus

582. Anterior axillary fold is formed by all of the following muscles **except**
    a) subscapularis
    b) pectoralis major
    c) pectoralis minor
    d) subclavius

583. Pectoralis major is supplied by the spinal roots
    a) c4 and c5
    b) c5 and c6
    c) c5, c6 and c7
    d) c5, c6, c7, c8 and T1

584. Axillary sheath is the tubular extension from
    a) clavipectoral fascia
    b) carotid sheath
    c) prevertebral fascia
    d) pretracheal fascia

Chapter V   Upper Limb 63

585. All of the following structures pierce the calvipectoral fascia **except**
   a) medial pectoral nerve   b) cephalic vein
   c) thoraco-acromial artery   d) lateral pectoral nerve
586. Cords of brachial plexus are named as per their relation with the axillary artery behind
   a) subclavius   b) pectoralis minor
   c) pectoralis major   d) deltoid
587. All of the following are attached to the coracord process of scapula **except**
   a) long head of biceps brachii b) coracobrachialis
   c) pectoralis minor   d) short head of bicepis brachii
588. All of the following muscles connect the ribs with the scapula **except**
   a) lattissimus dorsi   b) rhomboideus
   c) pectoralis minor   d) serratus anterior
589. Long thoracic nerve supplies
   a) lattissimus dorsi   b) subscapularis
   c) serratus anterior   d) teres major
590. Which of the following is a multipennate muscle?
   a) pectoralis major   b) lattissimus dorsi
   c) trapezius   d) deltoid
591. Which of the following structures lies in deltopectoral groove?
   a) brachial vein   b) cephalic vein
   c) basilic vein   d) axillary vein
592. Which of the following conditions simulates dislocation of shoulder?
   a) subacromial bursitis   b) acromial fracture
   c) atrophy of deltoid muscle   d) atrophy of pectoralis major
593. Lower subscapular nerve supplies which of the following muscles?
   a) lattissimus dorsi   b) infraspinatus
   c) teres minor   d) teres major
594. All of the following structures pierce the medial intermuscular septum of arm **except**
   a) superior ulnar collateral artery b) profunda brachii artery
   c) ulnar nerve
   d) posterior branch of inferior ulnar collateral artery
595. Lateral intermuscular septum of arm is perforated at the junction of upper and middle thirds by which nerve?
   a) ulnar   b) median
   c) musculocutaneous   d) radial
596. Which nerve traverses coracobrachialis muscle?
   a) axillary   b) musculocutaneous
   c) radial   d) ulnar

597. All of the following structures are related to coracobrachialis on its medial aspect **except**
    a) axillary nerve
    b) axillary artery
    c) axillary vein
    d) median nerve
598. All of the following are the actions of the biceps brachi **except**
    a) supination of forearm
    b) flexion at elbow
    c) flexion at shoulder
    d) it checks downward translation of humerus
599. The dislocated bicipetal long tendon from the bicipetal groove can be replaced by rotating the arm in and
    a) flexing the forearm
    b) extending the forearm
    c) flexing the arm
    d) abducting the arm
600. When long bicipetal tendon is dislocated from the bicipetal groove it fixes the arm in
    a) adduction
    b) abduction
    c) flexion
    d) extension
601. Which of the following muscles is attached to the ulnar tuberosity?
    a) supinator
    b) pronator teres
    c) brachialis
    d) biceps brachi
602. All of the following structures are anterior to brachialis **except**
    a) brachial artery
    b) median nerve
    c) biceps brachii tendon
    d) radial nerve
603. Muscle of arm supplied by nerves from both the compartments of arm is
    a) brachioradialis
    b) biceps brachii
    c) brachialis
    d) coracobrachialis
604. All of the following muscles are the flexors of forearm **except**
    a) palmaris longus
    b) brachioradialis
    c) biceps brachii
    d) brachialis
605. Muscle passing between teres major and teres minor muscles is
    a) subscapularis
    b) lattissimus dorsi
    c) short head of biceps brachii
    d) long head of triceps
606. Quadrangular space of axila transmits
    a) axillary artery
    b) axillary nerve
    c) circumflex scapular vessels
    d) axillary vein
607. Upper triangular space of arm contains
    a) circumflex humeral vessels
    b) circumflex scapular vessels
    c) suprascapular vessels
    d) profounda brachii artery
608. Lower triangular space transmits which of the following nerves?
    a) axillary
    b) ulnar
    c) median
    d) radial

609. Which of the heads of triceps is active in all forms of forearm extension?
 a) long
 b) medial
 c) lateral
 d) all three

610. When the arm is raised, the shoulder joint is supported from below by
 a) pectoralis major
 b) lattissimus dorsi
 c) long head of triceps
 d) long head of biceps

611. Muscle acting synergically to maintain semiflexion in forceful supination of a semiflexed forearm is
 a) triceps
 b) branchioradialis
 c) branchialis
 d) pronator teres

612. Nerve entering forearm between two heads of pronator teres is
 a) ulnar
 b) radial
 c) median
 d) musculocutaneous

613. Pronator teres muscle is supplied by which of the following nerves?
 a) ulnar
 b) musculocutaneous
 c) radial
 d) median

614. All of the following form boundries of cubital fossa **except**
 a) lateral margin of pronator teres
 b) medial margin of brachiordialis
 c) line joining the epicondyles of humerus
 d) tendon of biceps brachii

615. All of the following are the contents of cubital fossa **except**
 a) brachial artery
 b) median nerve
 c) ulnar nerve
 d) radial nerve

616. All forearm flexors are supplied by median nerve **except**
 a) flexor pollicis longus
 b) palmaris longus
 c) flexor digitorum superficialis
 d) flexor carpi ulnaris

617. Which of the following forearm flexors abducts the hand with radial extensors of forearm?
 a) flexor carpi ulnaris
 b) flexor digitorum profundus
 c) flexor pollius longus
 d) flexor carpi radialis

618. Tendon of which of the following forearm flexors passes superficial to the flexor retinaculum?
 a) flexor carpi ulnaris
 b) flexor digitorum superficialis
 c) palmaris longus
 d) flexor carpi radialis

619. Groove on trapezium bone transmits the tendon of
 a) palmaris longus
 b) flexor carpi ulnaris
 c) flexor pollicis longus
 d) flexor carpi radialis

620. Which of the following is the unipennate muscle?
    a) extensor pollicis longus
    b) adductor pollicis
    c) flexor pollicis longus
    d) brachioradialis
621. Muscle of forearm supplied by extensor compartment nerve but acting as flexor of elbow is
    a) biceps brachii
    b) flexor carpi radialis
    c) pronator teres
    d) brachiordialis
622. Which of the following nerves passes between the superficial and deep strata of supinator muscle?
    a) median
    b) anterior interosseous
    c) posterior interosseous
    d) ulnar
623. Supinator muscle is supplied by which nerve?
    a) ulnar
    b) median
    c) posterior interosseous
    d) anterior interosseous
624. In the lower forearm the abductor pollicis longus crosses all of the following structures except
    a) extensor carpi radialis longus tendon
    b) extensor pollicis brevis tendon
    c) brachioradialis
    d) radial artery
625. Which of the following arteries is the content of the anatomical snuff box?
    a) anterior interosseous
    b) radial
    c) posterior interosseous
    d) ulnar
626. All of the following structures pass through the carpal tunnel except
    a) ulnar nerve
    b) median nerve
    c) flexon digitorum profundus tendons
    d) felxor pollicis longus tendon
627. All of the following structures pass superficial to the flexor retinaculum of hand except
    a) ulnar nerve
    b) median nerve
    c) palmaris longus tendon
    d) ulnar artery
628. Flexor retinaculum of hand is attached to all of the following carpal bones except
    a) pisiform
    b) capitate
    c) scaphoid
    d) trapezium
629. All of the following muscles of polex are supplied by median nerve except
    a) abductor pollicis brevis
    b) adductor pollicis
    c) flexor pollicis brevis
    d) opponens pollicis
630. Which of the following palmar muscles is attached to skin?
    a) flexor pollicis brevis
    b) flexor digiti minimi
    c) opponens pollicis
    d) palmaris brevis

Chapter V

631. All of the following are the hypothenar muscles **except**
    a) flexor digiti minimi brevis
    b) adductor digiti minimi
    c) abductor digiti minimi
    d) opponens digiti minimi

632. Which of the following intrinsic muscles of hand link flexor to extensor tendons?
    a) dorsal interossei
    b) palmar interossei
    c) lumbricals
    d) thenar muscles

633. Which of the following interossei act as the abductor indicis?
    a) first dorsal
    b) second dorsal
    c) first palmar
    d) second palmar

634. Adduction of fingers is the movement of fingers towards the
    a) medial border of hand
    b) lateral border of hand
    c) index finger
    d) middle finger

635. Adduction of thumb is the movement of thumb
    a) towards the index finger
    b) away from the palm
    c) towards the palm
    d) away from index finger

636. Which of the following is not the hypothenar muscle?
    a) flexor digiti minimi brevis
    b) palmaris brevis
    c) extensor digiti minimi
    d) abductor digiti minimi

637. 'Intermediate palmar septum' of hand lies between the
    a) first and second lumbricals
    b) second lumbrical and flexor tendons of index fingers
    c) flexor tendons of index and that of middle fingers
    d) flexor tendons of middle and that of ring fingers

638. 'Middle palmar space' is limited dorsally by which of the metacarpals?
    a) first and second
    b) second to fourth
    c) third to fifth
    d) first to fifth

639. 'The middle palmar space' contains all of the following structures **except**
    a) deep palmar arch
    b) third to fifth digital flexor tendons
    c) second to fourth lumbricals
    d) digital vessels and nerves

640. All of the following lie in the 'thenar space' **except**
    a) tendon of flexor pollicis longus
    b) flexor tendons of index finger
    c) first lumbrical
    d) second lumbrical

641. Medial palmar septum is pierced by which nerve?
    a) muscular branch of median
    b) digital branches of median
    c) deep branch of ulnar
    d) superficial branch of ulnar

642. Which of the following nerves lies between the axillary artery and vein in axilla?
    a) musculocutaneous
    b) median
    c) ulnar
    d) axillary

643. Which of the following arteries gives rise to circumflex scapular artery?
    a) transverse cervical
    b) lateral thoracic
    c) superior thoracic
    d) subscapular

644. Pulsations of axillary artery can be better felt against which wall of axilla?
    a) medial
    b) lateral
    c) anterior
    d) posterior

645. Which of the following nerves lies on the medial aspect of the brachial artery in the cubital fossa?
    a) median
    b) ulnar
    c) radial
    d) musculocutaneous

646. Which of the following muscles form the floor of the cubital fossa?
    a) biceps brachii
    b) pronator teres
    c) brachialis
    d) brachioradialis

647. The ulnar head of pronator teres muscle separates the median nerve from
    a) radial artery
    b) ulnar artery
    c) radial nerve
    d) ulnar nerve

648. All of the following are the direct branches from the brachial artery **except**
    a) profunda brachii
    b) radial collateral
    c) superior ulnar collateral
    d) inferior ulnar collateral

649. Compression of brachial artery may be effected most favourably at
    a) its beginning
    b) its termination
    c) in the upper part of cubital fossa
    d) about midway in its course

650. Radial artery can be well palpated along the lateral border of tendon of
    a) pronator teres
    b) flexor carpi radialis
    c) brachioradialis
    d) flexor pollius longus

651. As the radial artery passes between the heads of first dorsal interosseous, it is crossed by the tendon of
    a) extensor pollicis longus
    b) flexor pollicis longus
    c) abductor pollicis longus
    d) extensor pollicis brevis

652. Which of the following arteries passes between the superficial and deep branches of the radial nerve?
    a) radial collateral
    b) radial recurrent
    c) radial
    d) ulnar recurrent

653. Which of the following nerves lies in the concavity of deep palmar arch?
   a) radial
   b) superficial branch of ulnar
   c) deep branch of ulnar
   d) median

654. Which is the main artery of superficial palmar arch?
   a) superficial palmar branch of radial
   b) deep palmar branch of radial
   c) superficial palmar branch of ulnar
   d) deep palmar branch of ulnar

655. Ulnar nerve lies on which aspect of the ulnar artery in the distal two-thirds of forearm?
   a) anterior
   b) posterior
   c) lateral
   d) medial

656. Ulnar artery passes posterior in its proximal half to all of the following muscles **except**
   a) palmaris longus
   b) flexor digitorum profundus
   c) pronator teres
   d) flexor carpi radialis

657. Common interosseous artery of forearm is the branch of which artery?
   a) ulnar
   b) radial
   c) brachial
   d) profunda brachii

658. Interosseous membrane is pierced by which artery in its distal part?
   a) common interosseous
   b) radial
   c) anterior interosseous
   d) posterior interosseous

659. Median artery of forearm is the branch of which artery?
   a) brachial
   b) ulnar
   c) radial
   d) common interosseous

660. Lateral cord of brachial plexus is formed by the
   a) anterior divisions of upper and middle trunk
   b) anterior divisions of middle and lower trunk
   c) anterior divisions of upper and lower trunk
   d) posterior divisions of all the trunks

661. Dorsal scapular nerve originates from
   a) lateral cord
   b) anterior division of upper trunk
   c) spinal root of C5
   d) upper trunk

662. Nerve to serratus anterior originates from
   a) spinal roots of C5, C6 and C7
   b) lateral cord
   c) upper trunk
   d) posterior cord

663. All of the following nerves are the branches from posterior cord of brachial plexus **except**
   a) upper subscapular
   b) dorsal scapular
   c) lower subscapular
   d) axillary

664. Nerve to subclavius muscle is the branch of
   a) spinal root of c5
   b) upper trunk
   c) anterior division of upper trunk
   d) lateral cord
665. Root value of medial cord of brachial plexus is
   a) c5, c6 and c7
   b) c6, c7 and c8
   c) c8 and T1
   d) c5, c6, c7, c8 and T1
666. Which of the following nerves supplies the rhomboideus muscles?
   a) thoracodorsal
   b) dorsal scapular
   c) long thoracic
   d) suprascapular
667. Long thoracic nerve supplies which of the following muscles?
   a) subscapularis
   b) lattissimus dorsi
   c) levator scapulae
   d) serratus anterior
668. Which of the following nerves is the branch from the upper trunk of the brachial plexus?
   a) dorsal scapular
   b) suprascapular
   c) long thoracic
   d) thoracodorsal
669. Which of the following nerves supplies the teres minor muscle?
   a) axillary
   b) thoracodorsal
   c) dorsal scapular
   d) suprascapular
670. Pseudoganglion ususally exists on nerve to
   a) supraspinatus
   b) teres minor
   c) subclavius
   d) lattissimus dorsi
671. Upper lateral cutaneous nerve of arm is the branch of which nerve?
   a) radial
   b) musculocutaneous
   c) axillary
   d) intercostobrachial
672. Which of the following nerves pierces the coracobrachialis muscle?
   a) axillary
   b) ulnar
   c) median
   d) musculocutaneous
673. Lateral cutaneous nerve of forearm is the branch of which nerve?
   a) musculocutaneous
   b) radial
   c) median
   d) ulnar
674. Intercostobrachial nerve communicates with which nerve?
   a) medial cutaneous nerve of forearm
   b) medial cutaneous nerve of arm
   c) ulnar
   d) median
675. Root value of median nerve is
   a) c6, c7, c8 and T1
   b) c8 and T1
   c) c5, c6 and c7
   d) c7, c8, T1 and T2
676. Nerve fibres joining the lateral root of median nerve to ulnar nerve are believed to be mainly motor to the
   a) flexor carpi radialis
   b) flexor digitorum superficialis
   c) palmaris longus
   d) flexor carpi ulnaris

677. Which of the following nerves proceeds in the forearm behind the tendinous bridge between the humeroulnar and radial heads of flexor digitorum superficialis?
   a) median
   b) radial
   c) ulnar
   d) posterior interosseous
678. Which of the following nerves is the largest branch of brachial plexus?
   a) axillary
   b) median
   c) ulnar
   d) radial
679. All of the following are the cutaneous branches of radial nerve **except**
   a) posterior cutaneous nerve of arm
   b) posterior cutaneous nerve of forearm
   c) lower lateral cutaneous nerve of arm
   d) lateral cutaneous nerve of forearm
680. Which of the following nerves shows the presence of pseudoganglion near its termination?
   a) anterior interosseous
   b) posterior interosseous
   c) superficial terminal branch of radial
   d) ulnar
681. Most frequently implicated nerve in the 'Crutch paralysis' is
   a) ulnar
   b) raidal
   c) axillary
   d) median
682. Damage to which of the following nerves causes 'Wrist drop'?
   a) radial
   b) ulnar
   c) median
   d) axillary
683. Which of the following vein is used most commonly for intravenous injection
   a) great saphenous
   b) median cubital
   c) basilic
   d) cephalic
684. The basilic vein pierces the deep fascia in the
   a) middle of forearm
   b) cubital fossa
   c) middle of arm
   d) axilla
685. Axial artery of the upper limb persists in the adult as the
   a) anterior interosseous
   b) posterior interosseous
   c) profunda brachii
   d) median
686. Interosseous recurrent artery is the branch from which of the following arteries?
   a) common interosseous
   b) anterior interosseous
   c) median
   d) posterior interosseous
687. Which of the following muscles is supplied by two nerves?
   a) pectoralis major
   b) supraspinatus
   c) deltoid
   d) biceps brachii

72 MCQs in Anatomy

688. All of the following muscles form the anterior wall of axilla **except**
    a) serratus anterior
    b) subclavius
    c) pectoralis major
    d) pectoralis minor

689. Which of the following muscles lie in the medial wall of axilla?
    a) pectoralis major
    b) serratus anterior
    c) subclavius
    d) subscapularis

690. All of the following bones take part in the formation of apex of axilla **except**
    a) humerus
    b) clavicle
    c) scapula
    d) first rib

691. At the level of which intercostal space in the nulliparous woman usually the nipples of the breast are placed?
    a) third
    b) fourth
    c) fifth
    d) sixth

692. Which of the following muscles is called as a 'Boxer's muscle'?
    a) deltoid
    b) serratus anterior
    c) quadriceps femoris
    d) biceps brachii

693. All of the following muscles form the posterior wall of axilla **except**
    a) subscapularis
    b) teres major
    c) long head of triceps
    d) lattissimus dorsi

694. All of the following nerves are the supraclavicular branches of the brachial plexus **except**
    a) dorsal scapular
    b) suprascapular
    c) thoracodorsal
    d) nerve to subclavius

695. All of the following muscles are supplied by the branches from the posterior cord of brachial plexus **except**
    a) lattissimus dorsi
    b) subscapularis
    c) teres minor
    d) serratus anterior

696. Which of the following nerves supply the teres major muscle?
    a) upper subscapular
    b) thoracodorsal
    c) lower subscapular
    d) axillary

697. 'Waiter's tip' position of hand is caused by damage to
    a) upper trunk
    b) middle trunk
    c) lower trunk
    d) ulnar nerve

698. Axillary artery ends at the level of
    a) insertion of coracobrachialis
    b) outer border of first rib
    c) inferior border subscapularis
    d) inferior border of teres major

699. Efferent lymphatics from the apical group of axillary lymph nodes unite to form which of the lymphatic channel?
    a) jugular
    b) right lymphatic duct
    c) thoracic duct
    d) subclavian

Upper Limb

700. First group of axillary lymph nodes to be involved in the hand infection is
    a) lateral
    b) posterior
    c) central
    d) apical
701. Enlargement of which group of axillary lymph nodes may obstruct the cephalic vein?
    a) lateral
    b) medial
    c) apical
    d) central
702. All of the following are the intrinsic muscles of the shoulder **except**
    a) deltoid
    b) serratus anterior
    c) supraspinatus
    d) subscapularis
703. Action of teres major muscle at shoulder joint is
    a) abduction and lateral rotation
    b) adduction and lateral rotation
    c) abduction and medial rotation
    d) adduction and medial rotation
704. Which of the following muscles is primarily responsible for maintaining the flexion at elbow joint?
    a) biceps brachii
    b) brachioradialis
    c) brachialis
    d) pronator teres
705. Which of the following muscles is mainly used while inserting a corkscrew?
    a) pronator quadratus
    b) pronator teres
    c) brachioradialis
    d) biceps brachii
706. Injury to musculocutaneous nerve in axilla will lead to loss of sensation on
    a) medial aspect of arm
    b) lateral aspect of arm
    c) lateral aspect of forearm
    d) medial aspect of forearm
707. Upper end of ulna gives attachment to all of the following muscles **except**
    a) pronator teres
    b) biceps brachii
    c) triceps
    d) brachialis
708. All of the following forearm muscles have two heads of origin **except**
    a) flexor carpi ulnaris
    b) pronator teres
    c) flexor digitorum superficialis
    d) flexor carpi radialis
709. Both the articulating surfaces in the acromioclavicular joint are covered by
    a) synovial membrane
    b) hyaline cartilage
    c) fibrocartilage
    d) elastic cartilage
710. Elbow joint can be described by all of the following terms **except**
    a) synovial
    b) complex
    c) compound
    d) hinge

711. Intertubercular sulcus of humerus contains all of the following structures **except**
    a) axillary nerve
    b) branch of anterior circumflex humeral artery
    c) long head of biceps brachii
    d) insertion of lattissimus dorsi
712. All of the following muscles help in abduction of arm **except**
    a) serratus anterior
    b) deltoid
    c) supraspinatus
    d) infraspinatus
713. All of the following muscles form the boundaries of quadrangular space of axilla **except**
    a) long head of triceps
    b) teres minor
    c) teres major
    d) short head of biceps brachii
714. All of the following form of boundaries of the lower triangular space of arm **except**
    a) shaft of humerus
    b) long head of triceps
    c) teres major
    d) pectoralis major
715. Which of the following nerves does not give any branch in the arm?
    a) radial
    b) musculocutaneous
    c) ulnar
    d) axillary
716. Which of the following muscles is inaccessible to palpation?
    a) coracobrachialis
    b) triceps
    c) subclavius
    d) supraspinatus

Chapter VI

LOWER LIMB

717. Disc between fourth and fifth lumbar vertebrae lies at the level of
    a) iliac tuberosity
    b) highest point of iliac crest
    c) tubercle of iliac crest
    d) posterior sup. iliac spine
718. Which of the following structures passes through the lesser sciatic foramen?
    a) sciatic nerve
    b) perineal nerve
    c) obturator nerve
    d) pudendal nerve
719. All of the following structures pass through the lesser sciatic notch **except**
    a) tendon of obturator internus muscle
    b) obturator nerve
    c) superior and interior gemelli muscles
    d) nerve to obturator internus
720. All of the following structures pass through the greater sciatic foramen **except**
    a) sciatic nerve
    b) femoral nerve
    c) pyriformis
    d) posterior cutaneous nerve of thigh
721. Following statements concering the pubic tubercle are correct **except**
    a) it provides attachment to inguinal ligament
    b) it can be palpated about 2.5 cm from the median plane
    c) it forms an important bony landmark in cases of inguinal hernia
    d) pubic tubercles of both side articulate to form the symphysis pubis
722. What type of joint symphysis pubis is?
    a) primary cartilaginous
    b) secondary cartilaginous
    c) synovial
    d) fibrous
723. Which of the following muscles act as a flexor at both hip and knee joints?
    a) gracilis
    b) sartorius
    c) semimembranosus
    d) rectus femoris
724. Which of the following muscles is attached to the iliotibial tract?
    a) gluteus medius
    b) gluteus maximus
    c) gluteus minimus
    d) quadriceps femoris
725. Which of the following muscles passes through the greater sciatic foramen?
    a) psoas major
    b) iliacus
    c) obturator internus
    d) pyriformis

726. Opening between the arcuate pubic ligament and the urogenital diaphragm in male transmits
   a) deep dorsal vein of penis
   b) dorsal artery of penis
   c) internal pudendal vessels
   d) pyriformis

727. Close-pack position of the hip joint is
   a) flexion, full adduction and medial rotation
   b) extension, slight abduction and medial rotation
   c) extension, abduction and lateral rotation
   d) flexion, adduction and lateral rotation

728. Which of the following is named as the 'Y-shaped ligament'?
   a) ischiofemoral
   b) iliofemoral
   c) pubofemoral
   d) transverse acetabular

729. The transverse acetabular ligament is the part of
   a) the ligament of femoral head
   b) iliofemoral ligament
   c) acetabular labrum
   d) fibrous capsule

730. Femoral vein is separated from the capsule of hip joint by
   a) pectineus
   b) psoas major
   c) adductor longus
   d) iliacus

731. Which of the following structures lies anterior to the tendon of psoas major in front of hip joint?
   a) femoral sheath
   b) femoral vein
   c) femoral nerve
   d) femoral artery

732. Nerve lying between iliacus and psoas major is
   a) lateral cutaneous nerve of thigh
   b) genitofemoral
   c) femoral
   d) obturator

733. Which of the following muscles cover the capsule of hip joint superiorly?
   a) pectineus
   b) rectus femoris
   c) psoas major
   d) pyriformis

734. All of the following muscles lie behind the hip joint except
   a) pyriformis
   b) gluteus minimus
   c) quadratus femoris
   d) obturator internus

735. Nerve descending most medially on the posterior aspect of capsule of hip joint is
   a) to quadratus femoris
   b) to obturator internus
   c) posterior cutaneous nerve of thigh
   d) sciatic

736. All of the following nerves supply hip joint except
   a) femoral
   b) obturator
   c) gluteal
   d) sciatic

737. When the thigh is flexed or extended with the foot off the ground
    a) the femoral head 'spins' in the acetabulum on transverse axis
    b) the femoral head 'spins' in the acetabulum on anteroposterior axis
    c) the acetabulum rotates on the femoral head in transverse axis
    d) the acetabulum rotates on the femoral head in anteroposterior axis

738. All of the following muscles are attached to the outer lip of iliac crest **except**
    a) lattismus dorsi
    b) quadratus lumborum
    c) tensor fascia lata
    d) external oblique abdominis

739. Anterior inferior iliac spine gives attachment to
    a) sartorius
    b) inguinal ligament
    c) tensor fascia lata
    d) rectus femoris muscle

740. The left iliac fossa contains
    a) vermiform appendix
    b) caecum
    c) end of the descending colon
    d) terminal ileum

741. All of the following ligaments are attached to the iliac tuberrosity **except**
    a) iliolumbar
    b) iliofemoral
    c) dorsal sacroiliac
    d) interosseous sacroiliac

742. Spermatic cord along its course crosses
    a) pubic tubercle
    b) iliopubic eminance
    c) pecten pubis
    d) symphysis pubis

743. Anterior surface of body of pubis bone gives attachment to all of the following muscles **except**
    a) pectineus
    b) gracilis
    c) adductor longus
    d) adductor brevis

744. All of the following structures are attached to the pecten pubis **except**
    a) conjoint tendon
    b) lacunar ligament
    c) pectineal ligament
    d) arcuate ligament

745. Nerve to obturator internus muscle passes out of the pelvic cavity through
    a) obturator canal
    b) femoral canal
    c) greater sciatic notch
    d) lesser sciatic notch

746. All of the following muscles are attached to the ischium **except**
    a) obturator externus
    b) quadriceps femoris
    c) semimembranosus
    d) semitendinosus

747. Angle between the transverse axis of head and that of the lower end of the femur is known as
    a) angle of femoral torsion
    b) angle of femoral inclination
    c) angle of obliquity
    d) none of the above

748. Direction of femoral head in anatomical position is
    a) upwards and anteromedially
    b) upwards and posteromedially
    c) downwards and anteromedially
    d) downwards and posteromedially
749. Angle between the neck and shaft of femur is approximately
    a) 25 degree
    b) 85 degree
    c) 125 degree
    d) 185 degree
750. All of the following muscles are attached to the greater trochanter of femur **except**
    a) gluteus maximus
    b) pyriformis
    c) gluteus medius
    d) obturator internus
751. Adductor tubercle of femur receives the attachment of
    a) gracilis
    b) adductor brevis
    c) adductor longus
    d) adductor magnus
752. A thin vertical plate of bone extending from the compact wall near the linea aspera into the trabeculae of neck of femur is
    a) intertrochanteric line
    b) intertrochanteric crest
    c) calcar femorale
    d) calcar avis
753. The only epiphysis in which ossification constantly starts just before birth is the
    a) distal end of humerus
    b) proximal end of ulna
    c) distal end of femur
    d) proximal end of tibia
754. The usual injury to the lower limb bones after the age of 60 years is
    a) fracture of the foreleg
    b) fracture of neck femur
    c) spiral fracture of shaft of femur
    d) tear of medial meniscus
755. In the anatomical position, the apex of greater trochanter of femur is on the line joining anterior superior iliac spine to
    a) pubic tubercle
    b) posterior superior iliac spine
    c) most prominant part of ischial tuberosity
    d) ischial spine
756. The largest sesamoid bone in the body is
    a) pisiform
    b) calcaneus
    c) femur
    d) patella
757. In the living, when standing, the apex of patella is
    a) at the level of tibial tuberosity
    b) a little proximal to the line of knee joint
    c) a little distal to the line of knee joint
    d) on the line of the knee joint

Chapter VI Lower Limb 79

758. The most anterior structure attached on the tibial intercondylar area is
   a) anterior cruciate ligament
   b) anterior cornu of lateral meniscus
   c) anterior cornu of medial meniscus
   d) posterior cruciate ligament
759. The posterior surface of medial condyle of tibia gives attachment to all of the following **except**
   a) capsular ligament
   b) medial patellar retinaculum
   c) semimembranosus
   d) tibial collateral ligament
760. Gap in the interosseous membrane between tibia and fibula proximally transmits
   a) anterior tibial vessels
   b) tibial nerve
   c) posterior tibial vessels
   d) common peroneal nerve
761. The proximal part of the medial surface of tibia gives attachment to all of the following muscles **except**
   a) biceps femoris
   b) semitendinosus
   c) gracilis
   d) sartorius
762. Groove on the posterior surface of medial malleolus of tibia transmits
   a) posterior tibial vessels
   b) flexor digitorum longus
   c) tendon of tibialis posterior
   d) tendon of flexor hallucis longus
763. Apex of medial malleolus of tibia gives attachment to
   a) flexor retinaculum
   b) deltoid ligament
   c) anterior tibiofibular ligament
   d) posterior tibiofibular ligament
764. All of the following bones are involved in the transmission of body weight **except**
   a) femur
   b) tibia
   c) fibula
   d) talus
765. The common peroneal nerve can be rolled against the
   a) neck of tibia
   b) neck of fibula
   c) lower end of tibia
   d) lower end of fibula
766. When the common peroneal nerve is pressed against the neck of fibula, it causes tingling sensation on the
   a) plantar aspect of foot and toes
   b) dorsal aspect of foot and toes
   c) lateral border of foot
   d) medial malleous
767. The apex of head of fibula gives attachment to which of the following muscles?
   a) gracilis
   b) semimembranosus
   c) semitendinosus
   d) biceps femoris

768. The posterior aspect of the lateral malleolus is grooved by
   a) tibialis posterior
   b) flexor hallucis longus
   c) peroneus brevis
   d) peroneus tertius

769. Which of the following ligaments is attached to the malleolar fossa of fibula?
   a) anterior talofibular
   b) flexor retinaculum
   c) posterior tibiofibular
   d) calcaneofibular

770. Regarding the union of epiphysis with diaphysis which of the following long bones show reversal of ossification pattern?
   a) radius
   b) ulna
   c) tibia
   d) fibula

771. The groove between the tubercles of the posterior process of talus contains the tendon of
   a) flexor hallucis longus
   b) tibialis posterior
   c) tibialis anterior
   d) flexor digitorum longus

772. Comma-shaped articular facet on the medial surface of talus articulates with which of the following bones?
   a) calcaneus
   b) tibia
   c) fibula
   d) navicular

773. Cuboid bone is grooved on its plantar aspect by the tendon of
   a) tibialis anterior
   b) tibialis posterior
   c) peroneus longus
   d) navicular

774. The navicular bone articulates with all of the following bones **except**
   a) calcaneus
   b) talus
   c) all cuneiforms
   d) cuboid

775. Which of the following metatarsals provides attachment to the tendon of peroneus longus?
   a) first
   b) second
   c) fourth
   d) fifth

776. Centres of ossification appear frequently before birth for all of the following tarsals **except**
   a) calcaneus
   b) talus
   c) navicular
   d) cuboid

777. Tendons of all of the following muscles may show the presence of a seasamoid bone **except**
   a) quadriceps femoris
   b) soleus
   c) peroneus longus
   d) tibialis anterior

778. Sesamoid bone is frequently seen in the tendon of which of the following muscles?
   a) flexor pollicis longus
   b) flexor carpi radialis longus
   c) palmaris longus
   d) extensor hallucis longus

Chapter VI   Lower Limb

779. All of the following muscles are responsible for abduction at hip joint **except**
    a) gluteus maximus
    b) gluteus medius
    c) gluteus minimus
    d) quadratus femoris
780. All of the following structures limit the abduction at hip joint **except**
    a) adductor muscles
    b) ischiofemoral ligament
    c) pubofemoral ligament
    d) medial band of iliofemoral ligament
781. All of the following muscles cause adduction at hip joint **except**
    a) adductors
    b) pectineus
    c) sartorius
    d) gracilis
782. All of the following muscles are the medial rotators of thigh **except**
    a) gluteus maximus
    b) gluteus medius
    c) gluteus minimus
    d) tensor fascia lata
783. All of the following muscles are the lateral rotators of thigh **except**
    a) obturator externus
    b) obturator internus
    c) quadratus femoris
    d) gluteus medius
784. Cogenital dislocation is most common at which of the following joints?
    a) shoulder
    b) elbow
    c) hip
    d) knee
785. In the dislocation of hip joint, the femoral head is usually displaced
    a) upwards
    b) downwards
    c) forwards
    d) backwars
786. Largest joint in the human body is
    a) shoulder
    b) elbow
    c) hip
    d) knee
787. The articular surfaces of knee joint approach congruence in
    a) full flexion
    b) full extension
    c) midflexion
    d) all of the above positions
788. Which of the following genicular nerves and vessels lie between the fibular collateral ligament and the knee joint capsule?
    a) inferior lateral
    b) superior lateral
    c) superior medial
    d) inferior medial
789. Oblique popliteal ligament of knee joint is derived from the tendon of
    a) popliteus
    b) semitendinosus
    c) semimembranosus
    d) biceps femoris
790. Tendon of which of the following muscles is intracapsular?
    a) semimembranosus
    b) popliteus
    c) semitendinosus
    d) biceps femoris
791. The lateral patellar retinaculum is angumented by
    a) iliotibial tract
    b) tendon of biceps femoris
    c) tendon of semitendinosus
    d) tendon of semimembranosus

792. Interval between the oblique popliteal and the fibular collateral ligaments is filled by
    a) iliotibial tract
    b) lateral patellar retinaculum
    c) ligamentum patellae
    d) anterior ligaments of fibular head

793. Which of the following describes the 'Coronary ligament' of knee joint?
    a) prolongation of iliotibial tract
    b) part of capsule between the attachments to meniscal rim and tibia
    c) fibrous extension from semimembranosus tendon
    d) fibrous extension from the sartorius tendon

794. The articularis genu muscle is inserted on
    a) ligamentum patellae
    b) patella
    c) tibial tuberocity
    d) suprapatellar bursa

795. Which of the following may represent the vestige of the inferior boundary of an originally separate femoropatellar joint?
    a) anterior cruciate ligament
    b) infrapatellar synovial fold
    c) posterior cruciate ligament
    d) infrapatellar bursa

796. Tibial collateral ligament is crossed superficially by the tendons of all of the following muscles **except**
    a) semimembranosus
    b) semitendinosus
    c) gracilis
    d) sartorius

797. All of the following statements regarding the menisci of knee joint are correct **except**
    a) these are the crescentic cartilage laminae
    b) their peripheral margins are thick and inner thin
    c) these are covered on both surfaces by synbvial membrane
    d) each covers about two thirds of its tibial articular surface

798. The lateral meniscus of knee joint is grooved posterolaterally by the tendon of
    a) lateral head of gastrocnemius
    b) biceps femoris
    c) semimembranosus
    d) popliteus

799. At the knee joint, when the foot is fixed, which of the following involves conjunct medial femoral rotation?
    a) full flexion
    b) full extension
    c) 30° flexion
    d) last 30° extension

800. Full flexion at knee joint including passive element occurs through
    a) 120°
    b) 140°
    c) 160°
    d) 180°

801. Close-packing position of knee joint is
    a) full flexion
    b) full extension
    c) mid flexion
    d) 30° before full extension

802. Unlocking of the knee joint with the foot fixed involves
    a) lateral rotation of femur during initial flexion from full extension
    b) medial rotation of femur during initial flexion from full extension
    c) lateral rotation of tibia during initial extension from full flexion
    d) medial rotation of tibia during last 30° extension
803. Which of the following is the unlocking muscle of knee joint?
    a) gastrocnemius
    b) semimembranosus
    c) popliteus
    d) biceps femoris
804. The line of body weight in symmetrical standing in relation to the transverse axis of knee joint is
    a) on the tansverse axis
    b) anterior to it
    c) posterior to it
    d) fluctuating
805. All of the following ligaments remain taught when the knee is flexed **except**
    a) fibular collateral
    b) anterior part of tibial collateral
    c) anterior cruciate
    d) posterior cruciate
806. Flexion at knee joint is checked by all of the following **except**
    a) anterior part of capsule
    b) fibular collateral ligament
    c) quadriceps femoris
    d) compression of soft tissues behind knees
807. Forward gliding of tibia on femur is prevented by which ligament?
    a) fibular collateral
    b) tibial collateral
    c) anterior cruciate
    d) posterior cruciate
808. All of the following can flex the knee joint **except**
    a) semimembranosus
    b) biceps femoris
    c) popliteus
    d) iliotibial tract
809. All of the following are responsible for medial rotation of flexed leg **except**
    a) popliteus
    b) biceps femoris
    c) semimembranosus
    d) semitendinosus
810. Which of the following muscles can cause lateral rotation of leg?
    a) biceps femoris
    b) popliteus
    c) semimembranosus
    d) semitendinosus
811. Proximal tibiofibular joint is what type of joint?
    a) syndesmosis
    b) symphysis
    c) plain synovial
    d) pivot
812. Which of the following ligaments of ankle joint is called as deltoid ligament?
    a) medial ligament of ankle joint
    b) anterior talofibular
    c) posterior talofibular
    d) calcaneofibular

813. Which of the following is the 'Close-packed' position of ankle joint?
    a) plantar flexion
    b) dorsiflexion
    c) eversion
    d) inversion

814. All of the following structures limit dorsiflexion at ankle joint **except**
    a) tendocalcaneous
    b) calcaneofibular ligament
    c) anterior talofibular ligament
    d) posterior fibres of deltoid ligament

815. All of the following muscles act as dorsiflexors at ankle joint **except**
    a) tibialis anterior
    b) tibialis posterior
    c) extensor hallucis longus
    d) extensor digitorum longus

816. All of the following muscles act as plantar flexors at the ankle joint **except**
    a) tibialis anterior
    b) tibialis posterior
    c) flexor hallucis longus
    d) soleus

817. The talocalcaneonavicular joint is what type of joint?
    a) saddle
    b) plane synovial
    c) pivot
    d) ball and socket

818. 'Inversion' is described as movement of foot in which the plantar surface faces
    a) forwards
    b) backwards
    c) laterally
    d) medially

819. Which of the following movements are associated with the inversion of foot?
    a) abduction and slight dorsiflexion
    b) adduction and slight plantar flexion
    c) abduction and slight plantar flexion
    d) adduction and slight dorsiflexion

820. Inversion of foot is checked by all of the following muscles **except**
    a) peroneus longus
    b) peroneus brevis
    c) peroneus tertius
    d) tibialis anterior

821. All of the following muscles limit the eversion of foot **except**
    a) tibialis anterior
    b) tibialis posterior
    c) extensor hallucis longus
    d) flexor hallucis longus

822. Which of the following muscles act as evertor of foot?
    a) tibialis anterior
    b) tibialis posterior
    c) flexor hallucis longus
    d) peroneus longus

823. All of the following muscles act as inverters of foot **except**
    a) tibialis anterior
    b) tibialis posterior
    c) flexor hallucis longus
    d) extensor hallucis longus

Chapter VI
Lower Limb 85

824. With the foot grounded, the body weight causes which of the following movements of foot?
   a) supination
   b) pronation
   c) inversion
   d) eversion

825. Lateral longitudinal arch of foot includes all of the following bones **except**
   a) calcaneus
   b) talus
   c) cuboid
   d) lateral two metatarsals

826. Which of the following is the main muscle supporting lateral longitudinal arch of foot?
   a) peroneus longus
   b) peroneus brevis
   c) tibialis anterior
   d) tibialis posterior

827. Which of the following is the main agent maintaining the transverse arch of foot?
   a) tibialis anterior muscle
   b) peroneus longus muscle
   c) long plantar ligament
   d) short plantar ligament

828. Flexor of thigh taking origin from the vertebral column is
   a) sartorius
   b) biceps femoris
   c) iliacus
   d) psoas major

829. 'Medial arcuate ligament' is the upper thickened part of fascia covering
   a) iliacus
   b) quadratus lumborum
   c) psoas major
   d) transverse abdominis

830. All of the following structures lie along the medial aspect of psoas major **except**
   a) femoral artery
   b) femoral vein
   c) femoral nerve
   d) pectineus muscle

831. Right iliacus muscle is related anteriorly to all of the following in iliac fossa **except**
   a) lateral cutaneous nerve of thigh
   b) terminal part of descending colon
   c) caecum
   d) terminal ileum

832. Which of the following structures lies anterior to the iliacus muscle in thigh
   a) femoral artery
   b) femoral vein
   c) femoral nerve
   d) profunda femoris artery

833. In symmetrical standing the line of body weight in relation to the transverse axis of hip joint lies
   a) far in front
   b) immediately in front
   c) on the axis
   d) immediately behind the axis

834. Which of the following muscles acts at both hip and knee joints?
   a) rectus femoris
   b) vastus medialis
   c) vastus lateralis
   d) vastus intermedius

835. 'Saphenous opening' lies about 3 cm away from the pubic tubercle
   a) superolaterally
   b) superomedially
   c) inferolaterally
   d) inferomedially
836. All of the following boundaries of saphenous opening are formed by the falciform ligament **except**
   a) superior
   b) medial
   c) inferior
   d) lateral
837. 'Falciform ligament' of saphenous opening is formed by
   a) superficial stratum of fascia lata
   b) deep stratum of fascia lata
   c) iliopsoas fascia
   d) inguinal ligament
838. All of the following structures pass through the saphenous opening **except**
   a) profunda femoris artery
   b) great saphenous vein
   c) superficial external pudendal vessels
   d) superficial circumflex iliac vessels
839. All of the following give attachment to tensor fascia lata **except**
   a) anterior 5 cm of outer lip of iliac crest
   b) superficial surface of fascia lata
   c) lateral aspect of anterior superior iliac spine
   d) deep surface of fascia lata
840. Nerve supply of tensor fascia lata is from which nerve?
   a) femoral
   b) lateral cutaneous nerve of thigh
   c) superior gluteal
   d) inferior gluteal
841. Which of the following is the longest muscle in the body?
   a) soleus
   b) sartorius
   c) flexor digitorum profundus
   d) sternocleidomastoid
842. The lateral boundary of the 'femoral triangle' is formed by
   a) the medial border of sartorius
   b) the lateral border of adductor longus
   c) the medial border of iliotibial tract
   d) the inguinal ligament
843. Which of the following muscles form the roof of the adductor canal?
   a) adductor longus
   b) sartorius
   c) adductor brevis
   d) gracilis
844. Which of the following nerves supply the skin of anterior 1/3 of scrotum?
   a) genital branch of genitofemoral
   b) femoral branch of genitofemoral
   c) ilio-inguinal
   d) perineal

Chapter VI Lower Limb 87

845. Which of the following nerves supplies the skin over the femoral triangle?
    a) femoral nerve
    b) ilio-inguinal
    c) femoral branch of genitofemoral
    d) obturator

846. Saphenous nerve is the branch of
    a) obturator nerve
    b) sciatic nerve
    c) common peroneal nerve
    d) femoral nerve

847. Skin of medial side of leg and foot is supplied by which nerve?
    a) sural
    b) superficial peroneal
    c) saphenous
    d) posterior cutaneous nerve of thigh

848. Which of the following artery crosses the spermatic cord anteriorly?
    a) internal pudendal
    b) deep external pudendal
    c) superficial external pudendal
    d) obturator

849. Which of the following muscles acts as a flexor at both the hip and knee joints?
    a) rectus femoris
    b) sartorious
    c) gracilis
    d) semitendinosus

850. Which of the following muscles acts as the extensor of thigh?
    a) quadratus femoris
    b) quadriceps femoris
    c) semimembranosus
    d) gracilis

851. Which of the following muscles is responsible for extension of leg?
    a) quadriceps femoris
    b) semimembranosus
    c) tibialis anterior
    d) extensor digitorum longus

852. All of the following heads of quadriceps femoris muscle take origin from femur **except**
    a) vastus lateralis
    b) vastus medialisq
    c) vastus intermedius
    d) rectus femoris

853. Which of the following adductor group muscles of thigh acts at both the hip and knee joints?
    a) adductor longus
    b) adductor magnus
    c) gracilis
    d) pectineus

854. Which of the following muscles is supplied by the obturator nerve?
    a) Sartorius
    b) semitendinosus
    c) biceps femoris
    d) gracilis

855. All of the following structures lie behind the pectineus muscle **except**
    a) adductor brevis
    b) psoas major
    c) obturator externus
    d) anterior branch of obturator nerve

856. Which of the following muscles is supplied by femoral nerve?
    a) pectineus
    b) gracilis
    c) obturator externus
    d) obturator internus

857. All of the following structures lie behind the adductor magnus muscle **except**
    a) posterior branch of obturator nerve
    b) sciatic nerve
    c) semitendinosus
    d) biceps femoris

858. Which of the following structures passes between the quadratus femoris and proximal border of adductor magnus muscle?
    a) nerve to quadratus femoris
    b) medial circumflex femoral artery
    c) inferior gluteal artery
    d) posterior division of obturator nerve

859. Which of the following muscles is supplied by nerves from two different compartments of thigh?
    a) rectus femoris
    b) gracilis
    c) adductor magnus
    d) biceps femoris

860. All of the following muscles are supplied by double nerves **except**
    a) brachialis
    b) adductor magnus
    c) soleus
    d) biceps femoris

861. All of the following muscles act as lateral rotators of thigh **except**
    a) gluteus minimus
    b) gluteus medius
    c) obturator externus
    d) obturator internus

862. Which of the following muscles is supplied by the inferior gluteal nerve?
    a) gluteus minimus
    b) gluteus medius
    c) gluteus maximus
    d) all of the above

863. Which of the following nerves lies between the gluteus minimus and medius?
    a) pudendal
    b) sciatic
    c) superior gluteal
    d) inferior gluteal

864. Which of the following muscles is partly internal and partly external in the osteoligamentous pelvis?
    a) obturator externus
    b) pyriformis
    c) quadratus femoris
    d) coccygeus

865. Inferior gemellus is supplied by which nerve?
    a) nerve to obturator internus
    b) nerve to quadratus femoris
    c) superior gluteal
    d) inferior gluteal

866. 'Trendelenburg's test' is positive in paralysis of which of the following muscles?
    a) gluteus medius and minimus
    b) gluteus maximus
    c) hamstring muscles
    d) quadriceps femoris

867. All of the following structures appear between the pyriformis and the superior gemellus muscles **except**
    a) superior gluteal nerves and vessels
    b) internal pudendal vessels and nerve
    c) posterior cutaneous nerve
    d) sciatic nerve
868. Which of the following nerves supply the pyriformis muscle?
    a) superior gluteal
    b) inferior gluteal
    c) branches from L5, S1 and S2
    d) nerve to obturator internus
869. All of the following structures lie on the medial aspect of the obturator internus muscle in the pelvis **except**
    a) obturator fascia
    b) levator ani muscle
    c) sheath of internal pudendal vessels and nerve
    d) obturator membrane
870. Which of the following nerves supplies the short head of biceps femoris muscle?
    a) femoral
    b) obturator
    c) tibial
    d) common peroneal
871. Which of the following structures lies along the medial border of the biceps femoris muscle?
    a) tibial nerve
    b) common peroneal nerve
    c) popliteal artery
    d) saphenous nerve
872. Tibialis anterior muscle overlies which of the following nerves?
    a) superficial peroneal
    b) deep peroneal
    c) tibial
    d) saphenous
873. Which of the following muscles act as dorsiflexor and invertor of foot?
    a) extensor digitorum longus
    b) tibialis anterior
    c) tibialis posterior
    d) flexor hallucis longus
874. Action of which of the following tautens the plantar aponeurosis?
    a) tibialis posterior
    b) gastrocnemius and soleus
    c) extensor hallucis and digitorum longus
    d) peroneus longus
875. Which of the following muscles is the part of the extensor digitorum longus?
    a) peroneus longus
    b) peroneus brevis
    c) peroneus tertius
    d) extensor digitorum brevis
876. Which of the following anterior crural muscles is supplied by the spinal nerve roots L4 and L5
    a) extensor hallucis longus
    b) tibialis anterior
    c) extensor digitorum longus
    d) peroneus tertius

877. The tendon of peroneus longus is attached to the
    a) dorsomedial aspect of fifth metatarsal
    b) lateral tubercle on the fifth metatarsal
    c) peroneal trochlea of calcaneus
    d) lateral sides of first metatarsal base
878. A second synovial sheath invests the tendon of which of the following muscles in the sole?
    a) tibialis anterior
    b) tibialis posterior
    c) flexor hallucis longus
    d) peroneus longus
879. Action of peroneus longus muscle on foot is
    a) plantar flexion and eversion
    b) dorsiflexion and eversion
    c) plantar flexion and inversion
    d) dorsiflexion and inversion
880. Which of the following muscles acts at both knee and ankle joints?
    a) soleus
    b) gastrocnemius
    c) tibialis posterior
    d) flexor hallucis longus
881. All of the following structures lie superficial to gastrocnemius muscle **except**
    a) plantaris muscle
    b) sural nerve
    c) peroneal communicating nerve
    d) small saphenous vein
882. Gastrocnemius muscle is supplied by which nerve?
    a) superficial peroneal
    b) deep peroneal
    c) saphenous
    d) tibial
883. What type of muscle the soleus is?
    a) unipennate
    b) bipennate
    c) multipennate
    d) circumpennate
884. 'Triceps surae' is formed by
    a) two heads of gastrocnemius and soleus
    b) two heads of gastrocnemius and plantaris
    c) soleus, tibialis posterior and flexor hallicus longus
    d) peroneus longus, brevis and tertius
885. The strongest tendon in the human body is
    a) tendon of biceps femoris
    b) tendon of tibialis anterior
    c) tendon of quadriceps femoris
    d) tendocalcaneus
886. In standing erect the centre of gravity in relation to the talocrural joint is on a vertical passing
    a) anteriorly
    b) through the joint
    c) immediately posteriorly
    d) far posteriorly
887. In erect standing the forward swaying at the ankle joint is overcome by the action of which muscle?
    a) tibialis anterior
    b) tibialis posterior
    c) gastrocnemius
    d) soleus

888. Which of the following muscles form the floor of popliteal fossa?
    a) plantaris
    b) lateral head of gastrocnemius
    c) medial head of gastrocnemius
    d) popliteus
889. Muscle acting only on knee joint is
    a) quadriceps femoris
    b) biceps femoris
    c) plantaris
    d) popliteus
890. With the foot on the ground, popliteus muscle rotates the
    a) tibia medially
    b) tibia laterly
    c) femur medially
    d) femur laterally
891. Which of the following muscles is said to 'unlock' the knee joint?
    a) plantaris
    b) gastrocnemius
    c) popliteus
    d) semimembranosus
892. Superolateral boundary of popliteal fossa is formed by
    a) semimembranosus
    b) biceps femoris
    c) medial head of gastrocnemius
    d) lateral head of gastrocnemius
893. What is the sequence of structures from before backwards in the middle of popliteal fossa?
    a) popliteal artery, vein and tibial nerve
    b) popliteal artery, nerve and vein
    c) tibial nerve, popliteal vein and artery
    d) popliteal vein, popliteal artery and tibial nerve
894. Tendon of flexor digitorum longus is crossed superiorly in the sole by the tendon of
    a) tibialis anterior
    b) tibialis posterior
    c) flexor hallucis longus
    d) flexor digitorum accessorius
895. All of the following structures lie superficial to the flexor digitorum longus muscle in leg **except**
    a) tibialis posterior muscle
    b) soleus muscle
    c) posterior tibial vessels
    d) tibial nerve
896. The distal attachment of the tendons of flexor digitorum longus is to the plantar aspect of base of
    a) the metatarsal
    b) proximal phalanx
    c) middle phalanx
    d) distal phalanx
897. Most deeply placed muscle in the flexor compartment of leg is
    a) soleus
    b) flexor hallucis longus
    c) tibialis posterior
    d) flexor digitorum longus
898. The direct continuation of tibialis posterior in the sole is attached to
    a) the sustentaculum tali
    b) navicular tuberosity
    c) medial cuneiform
    d) intermediate cuneiform

899. Which of the following structures lies behind the tibialis posterior muscles in leg?
   a) superficial peroneal nerve
   b) deep peroneal nerve
   c) peroneal vessels
   d) anterior tibial vessels

900. The main invertor of foot is
   a) tibialis anterior
   b) tibialis posterior
   c) flexor hallucis longus
   d) extensor hallucis longus

901. Tendon of which of the following muscles has a synovial sheath deep to superior extensor retinaculum?
   a) tibialis anterior
   b) flexor hallucis longus
   c) flexor digitorum longus
   d) peroneus tertius

902. All of the following structures lie deep to superior extensor retinaculum except
   a) superficial peroneal nerve
   b) deep peroneal nerve
   c) anterior tibial artery
   d) anterior tibial vein

903. Which of the following retinaculum of foot is 'Y' shaped?
   a) superior extensor
   b) inferior extensor
   c) superior peroneal
   d) inferior peroneal

904. Which of the following nerves supplies extensor digitorum brevis muscle?
   a) lateral terminal branch of deep peroneal
   b) medial terminal branch of deep peroneal
   c) superficial peroneal
   b) tibial

905. First layer of muscles of sole include all of the following **except**
   a) flexor digitorum accessorius
   b) flexor digitorum brevis
   c) abductor hallucis
   d) abductor digiti minimi

906. Which of the following muscles takes origin from flexor retinaculum?
   a) flexor digitorum brevis
   b) abductor hallucis
   c) flexor digitorum accessorius
   d) abductor digiti minimi

907. Abductor hallucis muscle is supplied by which nerve?
   a) superficial peroneal
   b) deep peroneal
   c) medial plantar
   d) lateral plantar

908. Which of the following muscles lies immediately superior to the central part of plantar aponeurosis?
   a) abductor hallucis
   b) flexor digitorim accessorius
   c) flexor digitorum brevis
   d) abductor digiti minimi

909. Tendons of which of the following muscles divides into two slips at the proximal phalangeal bases to accomodate another tendon?
   a) flexor digitorum longus
   b) flexor digitorum brevis
   c) flexor digitorum accessorius
   d) flexor hallucis longus

Chapter VI   Lower Limb   93

910. Tendons of flexor digitorum brevis are attached to
    a) the tendons of flexor digitorum longus
    b) the bases of proximal phalanges
    c) the bases of middle phalanges   d) the bases of distal phalanges

911. All of the following muscles are supplied by the medial plantar nerve **except**
    a) abductor hallucis   b) flexor digitorum accessorius
    c) flexor digitorum brevis   d) flexor hallucis brevis

912. Lateral plantar vessels and nerves are related to the medial border of
    a) flexor digitorum accessorius   b) abductor digiti minimi
    c) flexor digiti minimi   d) flexor digitorum brevis

913. Which of the following muscles is attached to both the processes of calcaneal tuberosity?
    a) flexor digitorum brevis   b) flexor digitorum accessoris
    c) abductor hallucis   d) abductor digiti minimi

914. Which of the following muscles belongs to the second layer of sole?
    a) flexor digitorum accessorius   b) flexor hallucis brevis
    c) abductor digiti minimi   d) abductor hallucis

915. Lumbrical muscles belong to which of the following layers of sole?
    a) first   b) second
    c) third   d) fourth

916. Tendon of which of the long muscles belong to the second layer of sole?
    a) flexor digitorum longus   b) tibialis anterior
    c) tibialis posterior   d) peroneus longus

917. All of the following lumbricals of the foot are bipennate **except**
    a) first   b) second
    c) third   d) fourth

918. All of the lumbricals of foot are supplied by the medial plantar nerve **except**
    a) first   b) second
    c) third   d) fourth

919. All of the following dorsal interossei are supplied by deep branch of the lateral plantar nerve **except**
    a) first   b) second
    c) third   d) fourth

920. Which of the following is known as a 'Shin bone'?
    a) femur   b) patella
    c) tibia   d) fibula

921. 'Pelvic girdle' is formed by
    a) two hip bones and sacrum   b) two hip bones
    c) one hip bone only   d) one hip bone and sacrum

922. All of the following muscles are attached to the pelvic girdle **except**
   a) psoas major
   b) iliacus
   c) sartorius
   d) obturator internus

923. A line connecting right and left posterior superior iliac spines passes through the spine of which vertebra?
   a) fifth lumbar
   b) second sacral
   c) fifth sacral
   d) first coccygeal

924. The tubercle of iliac crest is located on the outer lip of the iliac crest
   a) at the midpoint
   b) on the anterior superior iliac spine
   c) on the sloping posterior 1/3rd
   d) about 5 cm posterior to anterior superior iliac spine

925. With the hip bone in anatomical position which of the two bony parts lies in the same horizontal plane?
   a) anterior superior iliac spine and posterior superior iliac spine
   b) anterior inferior iliac spine and posterior inferior iliac spine
   c) ischial spine and superior end of pubic symphysis
   d) anterior superior iliac spine and pubic tubercle

926. A person's height is roughly four times the length of
   a) femur
   b) tibia
   c) humerus
   d) radius

927. Tibia articulates with all of the following bones **except**
   a) femur
   b) patella
   c) fibula
   d) talus

928. Most lateral point of the hip region is
   a) the greater trochanter
   b) ischial tuberosity
   c) anterior superior iliac spine
   d) tubercle of iliac crest

929. Small saphenous vein drains into which vein?
   a) great saphenous
   b) femoral
   c) popliteal
   d) tibial

930. The longest vein in the body is
   a) great saphenous
   b) inferior vena cava
   c) internal jugular
   d) cephalic

931. All of the following statements regarding the great saphenous vein are correct **except**
   a) it is the longest vein in the body
   b) it has 10-20 valves
   c) blood flows only from deeper veins to great saphenous vein
   d) it opens in the femoral vein

932. Which of the following nerves accompanies the small saphenous vein?
   a) saphenous
   b) sural
   c) peroneal communicating
   d) superficial peroneal

933. Which of the following vein is most commonly used for vein grafts?
    a) cephalic
    b) basilic
    c) great saphenous
    d) femoral
934. Which of the following nerves supplies the superomedial area of thigh adjacent to the scrotum?
    a) genital branch of genitofemoral
    b) femoral branch of genitofemoral
    c) ilioinguinal
    d) medial femoral cutaneous
935. 'Lateral cutaneous nerve' of thigh is the branch of
    a) lumbar plexus directly
    b) sciatic nerve
    c) femoral nerve
    d) genitofemoral nerve
936. All of the following muscles pass deep to the inguinal ligament **except**
    a) psoas major
    b) iliacus
    c) rectus femoris
    d) pectineus
937. Which of the following muscles is used to cross the legs in the tailor's squatting position?
    a) rectus femoris
    b) gracilis
    c) semimembranosus
    d) sartorius
938. All of the following muscles are supplied by the femoral nerve **except**
    a) sartorius
    b) iliacus
    c) rectus femoris
    d) tensor fascia lata
939. At birth, the patella is
    a) not present
    b) membranous
    c) cartilaginous
    d) bony
940. Patella becomes ossified
    a) before birth
    b) during first three years after birth
    c) during third to sixth year of life
    d) at puberty
941. All of the adductors of thigh are supplied by obturator nerve **except**
    a) pectineus
    b) gracilis
    c) adductor brevis
    d) adductor longus
942. Which of the following adductors of thigh receive double nerve supply
    a) gracilis
    b) adductor magnus
    c) adductor longus
    d) adductor brevis
943. The femoral pulse can easily be palpated 2 cm inferior
    a) and lateral to pubic tubercle
    b) to midpoint of inguinal ligament
    c) to midinguinal point
    d) to anterior superior iliac spine

944. Most of the blood to the head and the neck of the femur is supplied by which artery?
    a) obturator
    b) lateral circumflex femoral
    c) medial circumflex femoral
    d) inferior gluteal

945. All of the following structures are enclosed by the femoral sheath **except**
    a) femoral canal
    b) femoral artery
    c) femoral nerve
    d) femoral vein

946. The intermediate compartment of the femoral sheath contains
    a) femoral artery
    b) femoral nerve
    c) femoral vein
    d) lympatics

947. All of the following statements regarding the femoral ring are correct **except**
    a) it is the upper end of the femoral canal
    b) it is larger in females than males
    c) it transmits the lymphatics
    d) it is bounded laterally by lacunar ligament

948. Usually a femoral hernia can be palpated easily
    a) inferior to inguinal ligament
    b) at the root of scrotum/labium majus
    c) superior to pubic tubercle
    d) superior to midinguinal point

949. Which of the following arteries may be involved in strangulated femoral hernia?
    a) femoral
    b) obturator
    c) accessary obturator
    d) internal iliac

950. Which of the following canal is known as the Hunter's canal?
    a) femoral
    b) adductor
    c) pudendal
    d) axillary

951. Which of the following nerves accompanies the femoral artery in the adductor canal?
    a) femoral
    b) intermediate cutaneous nerve of thigh
    c) saphenous
    d) anterior division of obturator

952. Inflammation of popliteal lymph nodes is often due to lesion of
    a) lateral aspect of heel
    b) posteromedial aspect of thigh
    c) great toe
    d) front of knee joint

953. Lateral members of proximal superficial inguinal lymph nodes receive the lymphatics from
    a) external genitalia
    b) perineum
    c) gluteal region
    d) iliac region

Chapter VI Lower Limb

954. Medial members of proximal superficial inguinal lymph nodes drain the lymph from all of the following parts **except**
    a) upper part of uterus
    b) glans penis/clitoris
    c) lower vagina
    d) lower anal canal
955. Deep group of inguinal lymph nodes receives lymph from all of the following **except**
    a) testis
    b) glans penis/clitoris
    c) superficial inguinal lymph nodes
    d) lymphatics accompanying femoral vessels
956. Which of the following is the key muscle for understanding the relationships in the gluteal region?
    a) gluteus maximus
    b) piriformis
    c) obturator internus
    d) gluteus minimus
957. Longest nerve in the body is
    a) radial
    b) median
    c) vagus
    d) sciatic
958. The superior gluteal nerve is formed by the ventral rami of
    a) L2, L3 and L4
    b) L4, L5 and S1
    c) L5, S1 and S2
    d) S1 and S2
959. A single cutaneous nerve supplying largest area of skin in the body is
    a) lateral cutaneous nerve of forearm
    b) posterior cutaneous nerve of thigh
    c) saphenous nerve
    d) lateral cutaneous nerve of thigh
960. All of the following nerves supply structures in the gluteal region **except**
    a) sciatic
    b) superior gluteal
    c) inferior gluteal
    d) nerve to obturator internus
961. All of the following nerves arise from the anterior divisions of ventral rami of lumbosacral plexus **except**
    a) pudendal nerve
    b) nerve to obturator internus
    c) superior gluteal nerve
    d) nerve to quadratus femoris
962. Into which part of the buttock intramuscular injections can be given safely?
    a) superomedial
    b) superolateral
    c) inferomedial
    d) central prominent
963. Intramuscular injections in infants are given in
    a) gluteal region
    b) deltoid regin
    c) anterolateral region of thigh
    d) anteromedial region of thigh
964. The largest branch of the internal iliac artery is
    a) superior gluteal
    b) internal pudendal
    c) inferior gluteal
    d) superior vesical

965. 'Dorsal artery of penis' is the branch of
   a) superficial external pudendal
   b) deep external pudendal
   c) internal pudendal
   d) external iliac

966. All of the following are the contents of popliteal fossa **except**
   a) popliteal vessels
   b) great saphenous vein
   c) tibial nerve
   d) common peroneal nerve

967. The popliteal artery divides into its terminal branches
   a) in the adductor hiatus
   b) at the upper border of popliteus
   c) at the lower border of popliteus
   d) on the fibular head

968. Which of the following arteries accompanies the small saphenous vein?
   a) posterior tibial
   b) anterior tibial
   c) superficial sural
   d) inferior lateral genicular

969. Genicular branches for knee joint given by the tibial nerve are
   a) two
   b) three
   c) four
   d) five

970. Most commonly injured nerve in the lower limb is
   a) common peroneal
   b) femoral
   c) obturator
   d) tibial

971. 'High stepping gait' in a patient occurs because of damage to which nerve?
   a) femoral
   b) obturator
   c) tibial
   d) common peroneal

972. Loss of sensation on the sole of the foot is due to damage to which of the following nerves?
   a) superficial peroneal
   b) deep peroneal
   c) saphenous
   d) tibial

973. Nonunion of the fragments occur in the fracture of tibia
   a) at upper end
   b) through the nutrient foramen
   c) at lower end
   d) at the summit of middle and lower thirds

974. Skin on the dorsal aspect of first interdigital cleft of foot is supplied by which nerve?
   a) superficial peroneal
   b) deep peroneal
   c) medial plantar
   d) lateral plantar

975. 'Dorsalis pedis artery' is the branch of which artery?
   a) peroneal
   b) anterior tibial
   c) posterior tibial
   d) medial plantar

976. Common source of bone for grafting is
   a) radius
   b) ulna
   c) tibia
   d) fibula

Chapter VI

Lower Limb

977. In case of fibular bone transplant which part of fibula should be used?
    a) middle third
    b) upper third
    c) lower third
    d) any of the above

978. Which part of body of fibula is subcutaneous?
    a) upper third
    b) middle third
    c) lower third
    d) whole body

979. Talus articulates with all of the following bones **except**
    a) fibula
    b) navicular
    c) calcaneus
    d) cuboid

980. All of the following tarsal bones give attachment to muscles **except**
    a) calcaneus
    b) cuboid
    c) talus
    d) navicular

981. All of the following muscles are supplied by the tibial nerve **except**
    a) tibialis anterior
    b) tibialis posterior
    c) gastrocnemius
    d) soleus

982. Which of the following arteries lies in the lateral compartment of leg?
    a) posterior tibial
    b) anterior tibial
    c) peroneal
    d) none of the above.

983. Which of the following is known as the preaxial digit of lower limb?
    a) hallux
    b) little toe
    c) second toe
    d) middle toe

Chapter VII

THORAX

984. In pleural effusion, the level of pleural fluid is highest in
    a) midclavicular line
    b) anterior axillary line
    c) posterior axillary line
    d) midaxillary line
985. Which of the following spinal nerves is involved in the thoracic inlet syndrome
    a) first thoracic
    b) second thoracic
    c) seventh cervical
    d) eighth cervical
986. All of the following structures pass through the inlet of thorax in the median plane **except**
    a) oesophagus
    b) trachea
    c) left recurrent laryngeal nerve
    d) thoracic duct
987. Which of the following gives attachment to the suprapleural membrane?
    a) upper border of scapula
    b) posterior aspect of clavicle
    c) inner margin of first rib
    d) all of the above
988. The outlet of thorax is highest in which of the following lines?
    a) anterior median
    b) posterior median
    c) midaxillary
    d) midclavicular
989. All of the following diaphragms contain muscle **except**
    a) diaphragma sellae
    b) abdominothoracic
    c) pelvic
    d) urogenital
990. Structure lying behind the medial lumbocostal arch is
    a) vagus nerve
    b) lesser splanchnic nerve
    c) greater splanchnic nerve
    d) sympathetic chain
991. Upper limit of base of heart is marked by
    a) suprasternal notch
    b) sternal angle
    c) xiphisternal joint
    d) first costosternal joints
992. Costal margin is formed by which of the following cartilages?
    a) 10th to 12th
    b) 9th to 11th
    c) 8th to 11th
    d) 7th to 10th
993. The right posterior intercostal arteries pass behind all of the following structures **except**
    a) thoracic duct
    b) hemiazygous vein
    c) sympathetic chain
    d) oesophagus
994. Which of the following arteries are enlarged in coarctation of aorta?
    a) internal mammary
    b) subclavian
    c) anterior intercostal
    d) posterior intercostal

995. Which of the following posterior intercostal veins of left side drain into the accessory hemiazygous vein?
    a) 1st to 4th
    b) 2nd to 4th
    c) 5th to 8th
    d) 9th to 11th

996. Left second, third and fourth posterior intercostal veins drain into
    a) accessory hemiazygous vein
    b) hemiazygous vein
    c) azygous vein
    d) left superior intercostal vein

997. All of the following are the branches of internal thoracic artery **except**
    a) pericardiophrenic
    b) posterior intercostal
    c) superior epigastric
    d) musculophrenic

998. Which of the following nerves innervate the mediastinal pleura?
    a) vagus
    b) splanchnic
    c) phrenic
    d) intercostal

999. Which of the following vessel is related to the cervical pleura anteriorly?
    a) common carotid artery
    b) subclavian artery
    c) internal jugular vein
    d) internal thoracic artery

1000. All of the following arteries supply the parietal pleura **except**
    a) bronchial
    b) internal thoracic
    c) musculophrenic
    d) intercostal

1001. All of the following structures are related to the medial surface of the right lung **except**
    a) superior vena cava
    b) oesophagus
    c) thoracic duct
    d) trachea

1002. Which of the following structures is single at the root of each lung?
    a) bronchus
    b) bronchial artery
    c) pulmonary artery
    d) pulmonary vein

1003. All of the following anterior relations of the roots of lungs are common on both sides **except**
    a) phrenic nerve
    b) pericardiophrenic vessels
    c) anterior pulmonary plexus
    d) superior vena cava

1004. How much of the pulmonary area is occupied by the hilar shadows in PA view radiograph of chest?
    a) medial one fourth
    b) medial one third
    c) medial half
    d) medial two third

1005. Part of lung aerated by a respiratory bronchiole is known as
    a) a segment
    b) a lobule
    c) pulmonary unit
    d) alveolus

1006. All of the following are the components of a pulmonary unit **except**
    a) atria
    b) air saccules
    c) alveolar ducts
    d) terminal bronchiole

1007. Permanent overdistension of the lung alveoli is known as
   a) emphysema
   b) empyema
   c) pneumothorax
   d) dyspnoea

1008. During surgical resection of the bronchopulmonary segment the surgeon works to isolate a particular segment along the
   a) pulmonary arteries
   b) pulmonary veins
   c) bronchus
   d) bronchial arteries

1009. Which of the following structures run in the intersegmental planes of the lungs?
   a) pulmonary arteries
   b) pulmonary veins
   c) bronchus
   d) bronchial arteries

Chapter VIII

ABDOMEN, PELVIS AND PERINEUM

1010. Which of the following structures is retroperitoneal?
    a) duodenum
    b) ascending colon
    c) descending colon
    d) all of the above

1011. Which of the following structures have mesentry?
    a) ascending colon
    b) descending colon
    c) transverse colon
    d) kidneys

1012. All of the following structures have the mesentry **except**
    a) transverse colon
    b) small intestine
    c) sigmoid colon
    d) rectum

1013. All of the following are the peritoneal recesses present in the supracolic peritoneal compartment **except**
    a) right hepatorenal
    b) left hepatorenal
    c) right hepatophrenic
    d) left hepatophrenic

1014. Which of the following statements regarding the peritoneal cavity is true?
    a) It is communicated to the exterior in both male and female.
    b) It is not communicated to the exterior in both male and female.
    c) It is communicated to the exterior in males and not in females.
    d) It is communicated to the exterior in females and not in males.

1015. Lining of peritoneum is called as
    a) epithelium
    b) endothelium
    c) mesothelium
    d) any of the above

1016. 'Omental bursa' is the name for
    a) lesser omentum
    b) greater omentum
    c) lesser peritoneal sac
    d) greater peritoneal sac

1017. Gastrophrenic ligament is
    a) band of connective tissue between stomach and diaphragm
    b) double peritoneal fold connecting the stomach and diaphragm
    c) fibromuscular band of diaphragm extending to stomach
    d) none of the above

1018. Visceral peritoneum is derived from
    a) somatic mesoderm
    b) ectoderm
    c) endoderm
    d) splanchnic mesoderm

1019. Which of the following is the most complexly arranged serous membrane?
   a) pleura
   b) pericardium
   c) peritoneum
   d) tunica vaginalis
1020. Which of the following walls of the abdominopelvic cavity is firmly adherent to the parietal peritoneum?
   a) diaphragm
   b) posterior abdominal wall
   c) anterior pelvic wall
   d) posterior pelvic wall
1021. Peritoneum is most loosely attached to
   a) diaphragm
   b) posterior pelvic wall adjoining the rectum
   c) anterior abdominal wall adjoining the urinary bladder
   d) anterior abdominal wall above the umbilicus
1022. All of the following statements regarding the bare area of liver are true **except**
   a) it is devoid of peritoneal covering
   b) it lies between two layers of coronary ligaments
   c) its apex is formed by right triangular ligament
   d) its base is formed by left triangular ligament
1023. Regarding the peritoneal covering of the gall bladder which of the following statements is correct
   a) it is completely covered by peritoneum
   b) it is completely devoid of peritoneal covering
   c) its inferior surface and sides are covered by peritoneum
   d) its superior surface and sides are covered by peritoneum
1024. Attachment of lesser omentum on liver is to
   a) the fissure for ligamentum teres
   b) the fissure for ligamentum venosum
   c) the inferior margin of liver
   d) anterior surface of liver
1025. Which of the following is **not** contained in the free margin of lesser omentum?
   a) hepatic artery
   b) hepatic vein
   c) portal vein
   d) bile duct
1026. Which of the following does not form the boundary of the omental foramen?
   a) free margin of lesser omentum
   b) inferior vena cava
   c) quadrate lobe of liver
   d) first part of duodenum
1027. Peritoneum reflects forwards from rectum from
   a) the junction of upper and middle thirds
   b) the junction of lower and middle thirds
   c) the junction of sigmoid colon with rectum
   d) the anorectal junction

1028. What is the distance of the base of recto-uterine pouch (of Douglas) from the anal orifice?
   a) 10 cm
   b) 7.5 cm
   c) 5.5 cm
   d) 2.5 cm

1029. Which of the following structures in females correspond to the sacrogenital folds in males?
   a) broad ligament
   b) mesovarium
   c) marginal rectouterine folds
   d) none of the above

1030. Medial umbilical fold of peritoneum is formed by
   a) urachus
   b) obliterated umbilical artery
   c) inferior epigastric artery
   d) superior epigastric artery

1031. A fossa between lateral and medial umbilical folds is called as
   a) medial inguinal fossa
   b) lateral inguinal fossa
   c) femoral fossa
   d) umbilical fossa

1032. Appendices epiploicae are
   a) peritoneum covering the appendix
   b) peritoneal recess containing the appendix
   c) bands of longitudunal muscles of large intenstine
   d) small peritoneal appendages along the colon filled with adipose tissue

1033. The vermiform appendix frequently occupies which of the following recesses?
   a) superial ileocaecal
   b) inferior ileocaecal
   c) rectrocaecal
   d) intersigmoid

1034. The horizontal plane passing through the superior surface of body of the third lumber vertebra is
   a) subcostal
   b) transtubercular
   c) transpyloric
   d) transumbilical

1035. The transpyloric plane passes through the inferior border of which of the following lumbar vertebra?
   a) first
   b) second
   c) third
   d) fourth

1036. Which of the following transabdominal plane is situated midway between the jugular notch and pubic symphysis?
   a) subcostal
   b) transpyloric
   c) transtubercular
   d) transumbilical

1037. Transpyloric plane passes through all of the following structures **except**
   a) pylorus of stomach
   b) lower border of L-1 vertebra
   c) tips of eleventh ribs
   d) neck of the pancreas

1038. Aponeurosis of which of the following abdominal wall muscles form the inguinal ligament?
   a) transversus abdominis
   b) internal oblique
   c) external oblique
   d) all of the above

1039. Reflected fibres from the medial end of the inguinal ligament attached to the pecten pubis form
   a) conjoint tendon
   b) arcuate ligament
   c) reflected inguinal ligament
   d) crura of superficial inguinal ring

1040. Aponeurosis of which of following abdominal muscles splits to enclose the rectus abdominis muscle?
   a) external oblique
   b) internal oblique
   c) transversus abdominis
   d) all of the above

1041. Conjoint tendon of the anterior abdominal wall is attached to
   a) anterior superior iliac spine
   b) inguinal ligament
   c) pubic symphysis
   d) pecten pubis

1042. The most inferior aponeurotic fibres of internal oblique and that of transverse abdominis muscles form
   a) linea alba
   b) rectus sheath
   c) conjoint tendon
   d) inguinal ligament

1043. The lateral border of rectus abdominis muscle is known as
   a) linea semilunaris
   b) linea alba
   c) arcuate line
   d) linea gravidarum

1044. Which of the following abdominal wall muscles helps to stabilize the pelvis during walking?
   a) rectus abdominis
   b) external oblique
   c) internal oblique
   d) transversus abdominis

1045. Which of the following coverings of the testis is formed by the fascia transversalis of the abdominal wall?
   a) external spermatic
   b) internal spermatic
   c) cremastric
   d) Tunica vaginalis

1046. Neurovascular plane of the anterior abdominal wall lies between
   a) fascia transversalis and transverse abdominis muscle
   b) internal and transversus abdominis muscles
   c) internal and external abdominis muscles
   d) external oblique muscle and superficial fascia

1047. Cutaneous nerves to the periumbilical skin originates from the spinal nerve
   a) T9
   b) T10
   c) T11
   d) T12

1048. The lateral arcuate ligament giving attachment to thoracoabdominal diaphragm is the thickened band in the fascia on
   a) psoas major
   b) quadratus lumborum
   c) obliques abdominis
   d) erector spinae

Chapter VIII   Abdomen, Pelvis and Perineum   107

1049. The thick node in the diagonal band of the thoraco-abdominal diaphragm is in front of the
   a) foramen of morgagni
   b) aperture for inferior vena cava
   c) aperture for the oesophagus
   d) aperture for the aorta

1050. Which of the following arcuate ligaments is formed by the tendinous arch in the fascia of psoas major?
   a) median   b) medial
   c) lateral   d) all of the above

1051. Aortic opening of the thoracoabdominal diaphragm transmits all of the following structures **except**
   a) greater splanchnic nerves   b) azygous vein
   c) thoracic duct   d) aorta

1052. Oesophageal aperture in the thoracoabdominal diaphragm lies at the level of which of the thoracic vertebra?
   a) T6   b) T8
   c) T10   d) T12

1053. Which of the following diaphragmatic apertures lies at the level of 8th thoracic vertebra?
   a) aortic
   b) oesophageal
   c) inferior vena cava
   d) aperture for splanchnic nerves

1054. Apart from oesophagus, the oesophageal aperture in the diaphragm transmits all of the following structures **except**
   a) gastric nerves
   b) branches of left gastric vessels
   c) thoracic duct   d) lymphatics

1055. 'Prenico-oesophageal ligament' which connects oesophagus with the diaphragm is an extension of
   a) endothoracic fascia   b) fascia transversalis
   c) muscle of diaphragm   d) central tendon of diaphragm

1056. Opening for which of the following structures lies in the central tendon of the diaphragm?
   a) aorta   b) oesophagus
   c) inferior vena cava   d) thoracic duct

1057. Which of the following is considered to be the effective sphincter of the lower end of oesophagus?
   a) right crus of diaphragm
   b) left crus of diaphragm
   c) intrinsic muscle of oesophagus
   d) phrenico-oesophageal ligament

1058. Level of abdominal diaphragm is highest in
   a) supine position
   b) horizontal position on one side
   c) standing
   d) sitting

1059. Which of the following abdominal organs usually may herniate in the thorax?
   a) liver
   b) spleen
   c) right kidney
   d) stomach

1060. Patients of severe dyspnoea are most comfortable when
   a) lying down supine
   b) standing up
   c) sitting up
   d) lying down prone

1061. In adults, in quiet respiration tidal air inspired and expired in each cycle is about
   a) 50-75 ml
   b) 500-700 ml
   c) 5000-7500 ml
   d) 1200-1500 ml

1062. In quiet inspiration, the main and often sole active muscle is
   a) rectus abdominis
   b) diaphragm
   c) external intercostal
   d) internal intercostal

1063. Chief factor responsible for quiet expiration is
   a) diaphragmatic contraction
   b) anterior abdominal wall muscles
   c) elastic recoil of lungs
   d) intercostal muscles

1064. During forced expiration all of the following muscles contract **except**
   a) diaphragm
   b) external oblique abdominis
   c) transversus abdominis
   d) quadratus lumborum

1065. Dartos muscle of the scrotum is innervated by
   a) genitofemoral nerve
   b) pudendal nerve
   c) dorsal scrotal nerve
   d) ilioinguinal nerve

1066. In children, the testis can often be retracted in the loose connective tissue between
   a) superficial and deep layers of abdominal fascia
   b) deep layer of fascia and the external oblique aponeurosis
   c) the external and internal oblique aponeurosis
   d) transversus abdominis and the fascia transversalis

1067. 'Superficial inguinal pouch' in children lies between the
   a) external oblique and deep layer of abdominal fascia
   b) superficial and deep layers of abdominal fascia
   c) skin and superficial fascia
   d) external and internal oblique muscles

1068. Which border of the external oblique abdominis muscle is free?
   a) anterior
   b) posterior
   c) superior
   d) inferior

Chapter VIII   Abdomen, Pelvis and Perineum   109

1069. 'Popart's ligament' is synonymus with
   a) inguinal ligament
   b) lacunar ligament
   c) fundiform ligament of penis
   d) linea alba

1070. Which of the following is synonymus with 'falx inguinalis'?
   a) inguinal ligament
   b) conjoint tendon
   c) lacunar ligament
   d) reflected inguinal ligament

1071. Which of the following abdominal muscles form the bilaminar aponeurosis?
   a) external oblique
   b) internal oblique
   c) transversus abdominis
   d) all of the above

1072. All of the following are bilateral diagastric muscles of anterior abdominal wall **except**
   a) two internal obliques together
   b) two external obliques together
   c) two transversus muscles together
   d) one internal oblique with contralateral external oblique

1073. All of the following are the contents of the rectus sheath **except**
   a) superficial epigastric vessels
   b) inferior epigastric vessels
   c) rectus abdominis muscles
   d) pyramidalis muscle

1074. All of the following are the vestiges attached to the deep part of the umbilicus **except**
   a) ligamentum teres hepatis
   b) median umbilical ligament
   c) medial umbilical ligament
   d) lateral umbilical ligament

1075. All of the following structures form the anterior wall of the inguinal canal **except**
   a) superficial fascia
   b) aponeurosis of external oblique abdominis
   c) aponeurosis of internal oblique abdominis
   d) aponeurosis of transversus abdominis

1076. All of the following compose the fibrous sheet on obturator internus above the attachment of levator ani **except**
   a) pyriform fascia
   b) obturator fascia
   c) fascia of levator ani
   d) degenerated levator aponeurosis

1077. All of the following muscles compose the pelvic diaphragm **except**
   a) levator prostate
   b) puborectalis
   c) iliococcygeus
   d) sphincter urethrae

1078. Which of the following ligaments is commonly regarded as the degenerated part of the coccygeus muscle?
   a) sacrospinous
   b) sacrotuberous
   c) sacroilliac
   d) anococcygeal

1079. Muscle on the pelvic aspect of the sacrospinous ligament is
   a) pyriformis
   b) obturator internus
   c) coccygeus
   d) levator ani
1080. Pudendal canal is formed in which of the following fascia?
   a) obturator
   b) inferior fascia of pelvic diaphragm
   c) superior fascia of pelvic diaphragm
   d) superior fascia of urogenital diaphragm
1081. All of the following are the superficial perineal muscles **except**
   a) sphincter urethrae
   b) transverse pernei superficialis
   c) bulbospongiosus
   d) ischiocavernosus
1082. All of the following structures form the urogenital diaphragm **except**
   a) perineal membrane
   b) inferior fascia of levator ani
   c) sphincter urethrae
   d) deep transverse perinei
1083. Which of the following muscles is mainly responsible for maintaining penile erection?
   a) sphincter urethrae
   b) ischiocavernosus
   c) superficial transverse perinei
   d) deep transverse perinei
1084. Plane of inlet of lesser pelvis is bounded by all of the following **except**
   a) iliac crest
   b) sacral promontory
   c) pubic symphysis-upper border
   d) pubic crest
1085. In young adults the position of the umbilicus usually is level with the disc between
   a) T12 and L1 vertebra
   b) L1 and L2 vertebra
   c) L3 and L4 vertebra
   d) L4 and L5 vertebra
1086. Average capacity of stomach in adults is about
   a) 500 ml
   b) 800 ml
   c) 1000 ml
   d) 1500 ml
1087. The cardiac orifice of the stomach lies behind which of the costal cartilages?
   a) sixth
   b) seventh
   c) eighth
   d) ninth
1088. The distance of the cardiac orifice of stomach from the incisior teeth in adults is about
   a) 10 cm
   b) 20 cm
   c) 30 cm
   d) 40 cm
1089. All of the following ligaments are the continuous parts of the origional dorsal mesogastrium **except**
   a) gastrosplenic
   b) gastrophrenic
   c) splenicorenal
   d) gastrohepatic
1090. All of the following structures form the stomach-bed **except**
   a) left lobe of liver
   b) left suprarenal gland
   c) left kidney
   d) transverse mesocolon

1091. When the stomach is full, the lowest part is the
- a) pylorus
- b) pyloric antrum
- c) body
- d) fundus

1092. 'Steer-horn' type of stomach lies-almost
- a) vertically
- b) anteroposteriorly
- c) obliquely
- d) transversly

1093. Gastric canal of stomach extends from the cardiac orifice along the lesser curvature to the
- a) angular incisure
- b) sulcus intermedius
- c) pylorus
- d) middle of body

1094. Epithelium linning the oesophagus is
- a) stratified squamous
- b) transitional
- c) simple columnar
- d) pseudostratified columnar

1095. Lining epithelium of stomach is
- a) transitional
- b) psuedostratified columnar
- c) simple columnar
- d) simple cuboidal

1096. Which of the following cells predominate in the cardiac glands?
- a) mucus secreting
- b) zymogenic
- c) oxyntic
- d) entero-endocrine

1097. Which of the following cells are the source of gastric digestive enzymes
- a) zymogenic
- b) oxyntic
- c) mucus
- d) entero-endocrine

1098. Which of the following cells of the gastric glands are strongly basophilic??
- a) oxyntic
- b) mucus
- c) argentaffin
- d) peptic

1099. Which of the following cells of the gastric glands are known as parietal cells?
- a) oxyntic
- b) argentaffin
- c) zymogenic
- d) undifferentiated columnar

1100. Which of the following cells give beaded appearance to the gastric glands?
- a) argentaffin
- b) undifferentiated columnar
- c) zymogenic
- d) oxyntic

1101. Cells secreting hydrochloric acid in the stomach are
- a) oxyntic
- b) argentaffin
- c) zymogenic
- d) undifferentiated columnar

1102. Cells most numerous at the necks of gastric glands are
- a) mucus
- b) parietal
- c) cheif
- d) argentaffin

1103. Cells which rarely reach the lumen of gastric glands are
- a) argentaffin
- b) chief
- c) oxyntic
- d) mucus

1104. Which of the following cells secrete the intrinsic factor responsible for the absorption of vitamin B_{12}?
    a) argentaffin
    b) zymogenic
    c) oxyntic
    d) mucus

1105. Cells of the gastric glands with cytoplasm having strong affinity for silver salts are
    a) zymogenic
    b) argentaffin
    c) oxyntic
    d) undifferentiated columnar

1106. Part of stomach having gastric pits occupying about two-thirds of the mucosal depth is
    a) cardiac end
    b) body
    c) pyloric
    d) fundus

1107. The enteric hormone gastrin has been isolated from the
    a) cardiac glands
    b) pyloric glands
    c) main gastric glands
    d) all of the above

1108. Right gastro-epiploic artery originates from the
    a) coeliac artery
    b) common hepatic artery
    c) splenic artery
    d) right gastric artery

1109. Which of the following artery originates from the splenic artery?
    a) left gastric
    b) left gastro-epiploic
    c) right gastric
    d) right gastro-epiploic

1110. Which coat of the stomach contains a true plexus of arteries and atrerioles?
    a) serosa
    b) muscularis externa
    c) submucosa
    d) mucosa

1111. A portion of small intestine called as ileum is its distal
    a) one-fifth
    b) two-fifths
    c) three-fifths
    d) four-fifths

1112. Inferior duodenal flexure usually coresponds with the lower border of which of the following lumbar vertebra?
    a) first
    b) second
    c) third
    d) fourth

1113. Most mobile portion of the duodenum is its
    a) first part
    b) second part
    c) third part
    d) fourth part

1114. Duodenum is retroperitoneal **except** in its
    a) proximal half of superior part
    b) descending part
    c) horizontal part
    d) ascending part

1115. All of the following structures are related to the first part of the duodenum posteriorly **except**
    a) bile duct
    b) gastroduodenal artery
    c) portal vein
    d) quadrate lobe of liver

1116. Part of duodenum stained by bile after death is
   a) superior
   b) descending
   c) horizontal
   d) ascending
1117. Descending part of the duodenum is related anteriorly to all of the following structures **except**
   a) right kidney
   b) right lobe of liver
   c) transverse colon
   d) jejunum
1118. In the descending part of duodenum the major duodenal papilla is sited
   a) anteromedially
   b) anterolaterally
   c) posteromedially
   d) posterolaterally
1119. Anterior surface of third part of duodenum is crossed by
   a) inferior vena cava
   b) abdominal aorta
   c) superior mesentric vessels
   d) transverse mesocolon
1120. Posterior surface of the horizontal part of duodenum is related to all of the following structures **except**
   a) right ureter
   b) right psoas major
   c) right testicular vessels
   d) superior mesentric vessels
1121. All of the following arteries supply the duodenum **except** the
   a) supraduodenal
   b) pancreaticoduodenal
   c) right gastroepiploic
   d) left gastroepiploic
1122. Which of the following structures is almost absent from the proximal jejunum?
   a) circular folds
   b) aggregated lymphatic follicles
   c) villi
   d) all of the above
1123. Mesentry of small intestine crosses all of the following structures **except**
   a) right kidney
   b) right psoas major
   c) aorta
   d) inferior vena cava
1124. Mesentry between its two layers contains all of the followinbg structures **except**
   a) branches of superior mesentric vessels
   b) branches of inferior mesentric vessels
   c) lacteals
   d) lymph nodes
1125. Which of the following parts of the small intestine has the intestinal villi as broad ridges?
   a) proximal part of duodenum
   b) proximal part of jejunum
   c) proximal part of ileum
   d) distal part of ileum
1126. Which of the following parts of small intestine contain the branched tubuloalveolar submucosal glands?
   a) duodenum
   b) jejunum
   c) proximal ileum
   d) terminal ileum

1127. The epithelium of intestinal mucosa is mainly simple columnar **except** over the
   a) plica semilunaris
   b) intestinal villi
   c) lymphatic follicles
   d) intestinal glands

1128. Core of the intestinal villus contains all of the following structures **except**
   a) blood vessels
   b) lacteals
   c) non-striated myocytes
   d) lymph nodes

1129. Non-striated myocytes in the core of the intestinal villus clusters around
   a) arteries
   b) veins
   c) lacteals
   d) nerves

1130. The intestinal epithelium shows striated border appearance under microscope because of presence of
   a) cilia
   b) stereocilia
   c) microvilli
   d) all of the above

1131. The undifferentiated stem cells of the small intestine divide at the rate of one cell per
   a) 10 hours
   b) 100 hours
   c) 10 days
   d) 100 days

1132. Which of the following cells of the intestinal glands is rich in zinc?
   a) undifferentiated stem cells
   b) argentaffin cells
   c) zymogenic cells
   d) all of the above

1133. Which of the following cells of lining epithelium of digestive tract is classified as one type of the APUD cell?
   a) zymogenic
   b) oxyntic
   c) argentaffin
   d) mucous

1134. Ducts of which of the following glands of the digestive tract pierce the muscularis mucosae?
   a) gastric
   b) duodenal
   c) of ileum and jejunum
   d) of large instenstine

1135. Which part of the intestine shows presence of solitary lymphatic follicles in its wall?
   a) duodenum
   b) jejunum and ileum
   c) large intestine
   d) all of the above

1136. Which part of the stomach shows presence of the solitary lymphatic follicles in its wall?
   a) fundic
   b) body
   c) pyloric
   d) all of the above

1137. All of the following statements regarding the aggregated lymphoid follicles are correct **except**
   a) vary in length from 2-10 cm
   b) are most prominent around puberty
   c) are largest and most numerous in ileum
   d) villi are most numerous on its luminal surface

1138. Intestinal villi are usually absent in the ileum on luminal aspect of
   a) mesenteric border
   b) antimesenteric border
   c) aggregated lymphoid follicles
   d) circular folds
1139. In typhoid fever, ulceration of the aggregated lymphoid follicles of small intestine are
   a) oval across the long axis of gut
   b) oval, along the long axis of gut
   c) oval and oblique
   d) irregular
1140. Jejunal and ileal arteries are the branches from which of the following artery?
   a) abdominal aorta
   b) coeliac trunk
   c) superior mesentric
   d) inferior mesentric
1141. Lymph vessels are arranged in which of the following coats of the small instenstine?
   a) mucosal and muscular
   b) mucosal and serosal
   c) submucosal and muscular
   d) submucosal and serosal
1142. Ganglia present in the submucus and myentric plexuses of gut are
   a) parasympathetic
   b) sympathetic
   c) sensory
   d) all of the above
1143. Peristalsis of the small instenstine is generally augmented by stimulation of
   a) sympathetic system
   b) parasympathetic system
   c) both sympathetic and parasympathetic systems
   d) none of the above
1144. Parasympathetic stimulation augments all of the following **except**
   a) peristalsis of intestine
   b) intestinal secretions
   c) spincters
   d) anabolism
1145. Length of large intestine in human being is usually
   a) 0.5 m
   b) 1.5 m
   c) 3 m
   d) 6 m
1146. Diameter of large intestine is greatest
   a) at right colonic flexure
   b) at left colonic flexure
   c) in sigmoid colon
   d) near the caecum
1147. All of the following are characteristic features of large intestine **except**
   a) valves of Kerkring
   b) haustrations
   c) appendices epiploiae
   d) taeniae coli
1148. Three bundles of longitudinal muscles in the wall of large intestine are known as
   a) appendices epiploicae
   b) taeniae coli
   c) haustrations
   d) valves of Kerkring

1149. All of the following parts of the large intestine are devoid of appendices epiploicae **except**
   a) rectum
   b) sigmoid colon
   c) caecum
   d) appendix

1150. Which of the following parts of the large intestine is completely covered by the peritoneum?
   a) ascending colon
   b) transverse colon
   c) descending colon
   d) rectum

1151. All of the following parts of the large intestine show the presence of mesentery **except**
   a) appendix
   b) transverse colon
   c) rectum
   d) sigmoid colon

1152. Which of the following nerves is interposed between the caecum and the right iliacus muscle?
   a) femoral
   b) genitofemoral
   c) ilioinguinal
   d) lateral cutaneous nerve of thigh

1153. Which of the following is the frequent content of the retrocaecal recess?
   a) terminal ileum
   b) loop of ileum
   c) appendix
   d) lymph nodes

1154. Which of the following type of caecum is common in human being?
   a) infundibular
   b) quadrate
   c) ampullary
   d) intermediate

1155. Which of the following type of caecum represents the infantile form?
   a) ampullary
   b) quadrate
   c) intermediate
   d) infundibular

1156. Opening of ileum into caecum is located
   a) anteromedially
   b) posteromedially
   c) anterolaterally
   d) posterolaterally

1157. Intersection of right lateral and the transtubercular plane marks the surface projection of
   a) iliocaecal junction
   b) opening of appendix into caecum
   c) anterior superior iliac spine
   d) lower pole of right kidney

1158. Number of flaps of the valve of ileocaecal orifice are
   a) one
   b) two
   c) three
   d) four

1159. The valvular lips of the ileocaecal junction project into the lumen of
   a) ileum
   b) ascending colon
   c) appendix
   d) caecum

Chapter VIII Abdomen, Pelvis and Perineum 117

1160. Which of the following positions of the vermiform appendix is most common?
   a) pelvic
   b) retrocaecal
   c) subcaecal
   d) post-ileal

1161. Junction of the lateral and middle thirds of the line joining umbilicus and right anterior superior iliac spine is the usual surface marking for the
   a) base of vermiform appendix
   b) ileo-caecal orifice
   c) apex of vermiform appendix
   d) ileal diverticulum

1162. Which of the following caecal taeniea coli affords a guide to the appendix during surgery?
   a) anterior
   b) posteromedial
   c) posterolateral
   d) all of the above

1163. The length of human vermiform appendix on an average is
   a) 3 cm
   b) 6 cm
   c) 9 cm
   d) 12 cm

1164. Which of the followinng arteries gives rise to appendicular artery?
   a) right colic
   b) middle colic
   c) ileocolic
   d) inferior mesentric

1165. All of the following structures cross from behind the ascending colon **except**
   a) fourth lumbar artery
   b) ileoinguinal nerve
   c) femoral nerve
   d) iliohypogastric nerve

1166. All of the following structures lie above the transverse colon **except**
   a) liver
   b) gall bladder
   c) spleen
   d) head of the pancreas

1167. All of the following are the posterior relations of the transverse colon **except**
   a) head of pancreas
   b) descending part of duodenum
   c) upper end of the mesentry
   d) spleen

1168. Phrenicocolic ligament attaches the diaphragm to the
   a) ascending colon
   b) right colic flexure
   c) left colic flexure
   d) transverse colon

1169. Which of the following parts of the colon is longest?
   a) ascending
   b) transverse
   c) descending
   d) sigmoid

1170. Which of the following structure/s cross/ess the descending but not the ascending colon from behind?
   a) femoral nerve
   b) genitofemoral nerve
   c) vessels/gonadal
   d) all of the above

1171. All of the following structures lie posterior to the sigmoid colon **except**
   a) left ureter
   b) left ductus deference
   c) left internal iliac vessels
   d) pyriformis

1172. At the level of which of the sacral vertebra the sigmoid colon is continuous with the rectum?
   a) first
   b) second
   c) third
   d) fourth

1173. Anorectal junction lies at the level of
   a) fourth sacral vertebra
   b) fifth sacral vertebra
   c) tip of the coccyx
   d) slightly below the tip of coccyx

1174. Which of the lateral curves of rectum is convex to the left?
   a) upper
   b) lower
   c) middle
   d) upper and lower both

1175. Which of the following features of the sigmoid colon is present in the rectum?
   a) appendices epiploicae
   b) taeniae coli
   c) haustrations
   d) mesentry

1176. Which of the following parts of the rectum are covered by the peritoneum in front?
   a) upper third
   b) middle third
   c) upper two-thirds
   d) whole length

1177. The distance of rectouterine pouch from the anus in female is about
   a) 5.5 cm
   b) 7.5 cm
   c) 9.5 cm
   d) 11.5 cm

1178. Which of the following bend of rectum is termed as the perineal flexure?
   a) anteroposterior sacrococcygeal
   b) middle lateral
   c) lower lateral
   d) backward bent at anorectal junction

1179. Which of the following muscosal folds of the rectum are effaced during its distention?
   a) longitudinal
   b) horizontal
   c) both
   d) none

1180. Circular muscle is more prominant in which of the following horizontal mucosal folds of the rectum?
   a) upper
   b) middle
   c) lower
   d) all of the above

1181. Which of the following horizontal mucosal folds of the rectum projects just below the anterior peritoneal reflection?
   a) upper
   b) middle
   c) lower
   d) none

Chapter VIII — Abdomen, Pelvis and Perineum

1182. Which part of the rectum is normally empty **except** during defaecation?
   a) upper third
   b) upper two thirds
   c) whole
   d) below the middle horizontal fold

1183. Part of the rectum derived from the cloaca is
   a) whole
   b) upper third
   c) below the horizontal middle fold
   d) above the horizontal middle fold

1184. All of the following structures lie posterior to the rectum in the median plane **except**
   a) coccyx
   b) median sacral vessels
   c) ganglion impar
   d) sympathetic chain

1185. The fibro-areolar tissue connecting the rectum along the lines of anterior sacral foramina encloses all of the following structures **except**
   a) rami of superior rectal vessels
   b) lymph nodes
   c) dorsal rami of sacral nerves
   d) pelvic splanchnic neves

1186. Anterior to the rectum in males, **below** the reflexion of peritoneum all of the following structures are related **except**
   a) coils of ileum
   b) base of urinary bladder
   c) terminal parts of ureters
   d) ductus deference

1187. Length of anal canal in adults is about
   a) 4 cm
   b) 6 cm
   c) 8 cm
   d) 10 cm

1188. The terminal radicles of the superior rectal vessels are large in all of the 'anal columns' **except**
   a) left lateral
   b) left anterior
   c) right anterior
   d) right posterior

1189. Enlargement of venous radicals in which of the following anal columns constitute primary internal haemorrhoids?
   a) right anterior
   b) right posterior
   c) left lateral
   d) all of the above

1190. Anal sinuses are deepest in which wall of the anal canal?
   a) anterior
   b) posterior
   c) medial
   d) lateral

1191. Which of the following corresponds with the site of anal membrane in early foetal life?
   a) pectinate line
   b) site of attachment of anal valves
   c) middle of sphincter ani internus
   d) all of the above

1192. Which of the following represent the junction of ectodermal and endodermal parts of the anal canal?
   a) white line
   b) pectinate line
   c) anorectal junction
   d) none of the above

1193. Which of the following is the endodermal part of the anal canal?
   a) whole of it
   b) above the white line
   c) above the pectinate line
   d) between pectinate line and lower end

1194. Part of the anal canal lined by the nonkeratinized stratified squamous epithelium is
   a) above the pectinate line
   b) pecten
   c) whole of it
   d) below the white line

1195. All of the following statements regarding the white line of Hilton in anal canal are correct **except**
   a) it separates simple columnar from stratified squamous epithelium
   b) it is bluish pink in colour
   c) it is at a level between the subcutaneous part of external sphincter and lower border of internal sphincter
   d) digital examination reveals an anal intersphincteric groove at this site.

1196. A small depression receiving the opening of the ducts of anal glands is termed as the
   a) anal column
   b) anal fistula
   c) anal crypt
   d) anal sinus

1197. Which of the following structures of anal canal is lined by stratified columnar epithelium?
   a) part above the pectinate line
   b) part below the white line
   c) pecten
   d) anal glands

1198. Spincter ani internus ends below around the anus at the level of the
   a) pectinate line
   b) white line
   c) anorectal junction
   d) lower end of anal canal

1199. Which of the following parts of the sphincter ani externus lies horizontally below the lower borders of internal sphincter?
   a) superficial
   b) subcutaneous
   c) deep
   d) all of the above

1200. Which of the following parts of the sphincter ani externus is attached to bone?
   a) superficial
   b) subcutaneous
   c) deep
   d) none of the above

1201. Which of the anal sphincter can be voluntarily contracted?
   a) internal
   b) external
   c) both of the above
   d) none

Chapter VIII
Abdomen, Pelvis and Perineum 121

1202. The conjoint longitudinal coat of the anal canal breaks up into circumferential septa at the level of
    a) anorectal junction
    b) pectinate line
    c) white line of Hilton
    d) terminal end of anal canal

1203. The circumferential septa of the conjoint longitudinal coat of the anal canal are largely
    a) collagen fibres
    b) elastic fibres
    c) non-striated muscle fibres
    d) striated muscle fibres

1204. The anal intersphincteric groove corresponds with the
    a) anorectal junction
    b) terminal end of anal canal
    c) pectinate line
    d) white line

1205. 'Corrugator cutis ani' muscle is derived mainly from the
    a) conjoint longitudinal coat
    b) circular muscle of anal canal
    c) internal sphincter muscle
    d) external sphincter muscle

1206. All of the following muscles form the anorectal ring **except**
    a) puborectalis
    b) deep external sphincter
    c) internal sphincter
    d) conjoint longitudinal coat

1207. 'Fissure in ano' is very painful because it involves the
    a) lower dermal part of anal canal
    b) mucosal part of anal canal
    c) mucosal part of rectum
    d) mucosal part of rectum and anal canal

1208. During per rectal examination, the first resistance felt is because of
    a) superficial part fo external sphincter
    b) internal sphinter
    c) deep part of external sphincter
    d) subcutaneous part of external sphincter

1209. Which of the following vessels are contained in the lateral rectal ligaments?
    a) superior
    b) middle
    c) inferior
    d) all of the above

1210. The pelvirectal space is divided into anterior and posterior by the
    a) lateral rectal ligament
    b) fascia of Waldeyer
    c) rectovesical fascia
    d) pyriform fascia

1211. Fat-filled projections of peritoneum on the outer aspect of large intenstine are termed as
    a) taeniae coli
    b) haustrations
    c) appendices epiploicae
    d) sacculations

1212. Middle rectal artery is the branch of which of the following arteries?
    a) superior mesentric
    b) inferior mesentric
    c) internal iliac
    d) external iliac

1213. Which of the following arteries gives rise to inferior rectal artery?
   a) internal pudendal
   b) internal iliac
   c) superior mesentric
   d) inferior mesentric

1214. Which of the following arteries supplies the posterior part of the anorectal junction and that of anal canal?
   a) superior rectal
   b) inferior rectal
   c) middle rectal
   d) median sacral

1215. Which of the following arteries of rectum originates from the internal iliac artery?
   a) superior rectal
   b) middle rectal
   c) inferior rectal
   d) median sacral

1216. Indirect inguinal herina ememrging at the superficial inguinal ring is invested by which of the following structure?
   a) internal spermatic fascia
   b) cremasteric fascia
   c) external spermatic fascia
   d) all of the above

1217. In the complete congenital inguinal hernia, the herniated structure passes through the deep inguinal ring
   a) but not beyond the superficial inguinal ring
   b) upto root of the scrotum
   c) upto the upper pole of testis
   d) into the tunica vaginalis

1218. In the surgery of the strangulated oblique inguinal herina the deep inguinal ring should be cut
   a) superolaterally
   b) inferolaterally
   c) superomedially
   d) inferomedially

1219. The obliteration of the processuss vaginalis at birth starts and extends to opposite end to complete the fibrosis from
   a) superficial inguinal ring
   b) deep inguinal ring
   c) deep inguinal ring and head of the epididymis
   d) superficial inguinal ring and the head of the epididymis

1220. Which of the following does not form the boundary of the inguinal triangle?
   a) lateral border of pyramidalis
   b) lateral border of rectus abdominis
   c) medial half of inguinal ligament
   d) inferior epigastric artery

1221. The direct inguinal hernia occuring through the medial inguinal fossa lies between which layers of the spermatic cord?
   a) inside internal spermatic fascia
   b) between internal spermatic and cremasteric fascia
   c) between cremasteric and external spermatic fascia
   d) outside the external spermatic fascia

222. The direct inguinal hernia through the medial inguinal fossa is
   a) lateral to of inguinal canal
   b) lateral to conjoint tendon
   c) medial to conjoint tendon
   d) medial to lateral border of rectus abdominis

223. Which of the following is the common covering in all the varieties of the inguinal hernia?
   a) internal spermatic fascia
   b) fascia transversalis
   c) cremasteric fascia
   d) external spermatic fascia

224. Which of the following inguinal hernias shares all the coverings of the spermatic cord?
   a) oblique
   b) direct lateral
   c) direct medial
   d) all of the above

225. Which of the following inguinal hernias lies lateral to the inferior epigastric artery?
   a) indirect
   b) direct lateral
   c) direct medial
   d) all of the above

226. Which of the following inguinal hernia is called as bubonocele?
   a) incomplete indirect
   b) complete indirect
   c) medial direct
   d) lateral direct

227. Which of the following hernias is most common in young adults?
   a) oblique
   b) lateral direct
   c) medial direct
   d) umbilical

228. All of the following are the main pecularities of the direct inguinal hernia except
   a) it traverses the inguinal canal
   b) it is sited above the body of pubic bone
   c) the inferior epigastric artery is lateral to the neck of its sac
   d) the spermatic cord is posterolateral to it

229. All of the following are the coverings of the femoral hernia except
   a) peritoneum
   b) fascia transversalis
   c) femoral septum
   d) femoral sheath

230. Which of the following is the most important landmark in distinguishing inguinal from femoral hernias?
   a) superficial inguinal ring
   b) midinguinal point
   c) pubic tubercle
   d) inguinal ligament

231. Which of the following type of the umbilical hernias is due to failure of retraction of the umbilical loop of gut?
   a) infantile
   b) congenital
   c) acquired
   d) all of the above

232. Splenorenal ligament contains all of the following structures except
   a) renal vein
   b) splenic artery
   c) splenic vein
   d) tail of pancreas

1233. Uncinate process of the pancreas lies
   a) in front of superior mesentric vessels
   b) behind superior mesentric vessels
   c) behind gastroduodenal artery
   d) in front of gastroduodenal artery

1234. Anteriorly, the groove between head and neck of pancreas contains
   a) gastroduodenal artery
   b) superior mesentric vein
   c) splenic vein
   d) inferior mesentric vein

1235. Portal vein is formed by union of which of the following veins?
   a) superior and inferior mesentric
   b) superior mesentric and splenic
   c) superior mesentric and gastroduodenal
   d) inferior mesentric and splenic

1236. The uncinate process of the pancreas is crossed in front by the
   a) splenic vessels
   b) portal vein
   c) superior mesentric vessels
   d) inferior mesentric vessels

1237. All of the following are the anterior relations of the neck of pancreas except
   a) pylorus
   b) gastroduodenal artery
   c) anterior superior pancreaticoduodenal artery
   d) inferior mesentric vein

1238. Projection from the right end of superior border of the pancreas is known as
   a) omental bursa
   b) omental tuberosity
   c) uncinate process
   d) none of the above

1239. Two layers of the transverse mesocolon diverge from which of the following borders of the pancreas?
   a) superior
   b) anterior
   c) inferior
   d) none of the above

1240. Which of the following gland shows the presence of centro-acinar cells?
   a) mammary   b) prostate   c) parotid   d) pancreas

1241. Exocrine part of the pancreas secretes
   a) mucous secretion
   b) serous secretion
   c) seromucous mixed secretion
   d) hormones

1242. Islets of Langerhans are most numerous in which part of pancreas?
   a) head
   b) body
   c) uncinate process
   d) tail

1243. Which of the following cells of islets of Langerhans secrete the hormone glucagon?
   a) alpha
   b) beta
   c) delta
   d) peptide secreting (PP)

Chapter VIII   Abdomen, Pelvis and Perineum   125

244. Which of the following cells tend to be more central in the 'islets of Langerhans'?
 a) alpha
 b) beta
 c) delta
 d) peptide secreting

245. D cells, discovered in the human islets of Langerhans, are said to secrete
 a) gastrin
 b) glucagon
 c) insulin
 d) all of the above

246. Which of the following cells are not restricted to the islets, being also scattered throughout the exocrine tissue of pancreas?
 a) alpha
 b) beta
 c) delta
 d) peptide-secreting

247. All of the following veins drain the pancreas **except**
 a) superior mesentric
 b) inferior mesentric
 c) splenic
 d) portal

248. Nerve supply to the pancreas is from which of the following plexus?
 a) coeliac
 b) superior mesentric
 c) inferior mesentric
 d) all of the above

1249. The parasympathetic postganglionic neurons supplying the pancreas are located
 a) in the inter- and intralobular connective tissue
 b) in the inferior vagal ganglia
 c) on the wall of duodenum
 d) in the coeliac ganglia

1250. Pancreatic cysts usually push
 a) forwards
 b) backwards
 c) upwards
 d) downwars

1251. Carcinoma of pancreas usually affects its
 a) tail
 b) body
 c) head
 d) uncinate process

1252. Normally the liver occupies all of the following abdominal areas **except**
 a) right hypochondriac
 b) right lumbar
 c) epigastric
 d) left hypochondriac

1253. The average weight of liver in the males is about
 a) 0.5 kg
 b) 1.5 kg
 c) 3.5 kg
 d) 5 kg

1254. Which of the following parts of the liver is not served by the right hepatic duct?
 a) caudate lobe
 b) caudate process
 c) quadrate lobe
 d) right lobe

1255. The fissure for ligamentum venosum contains two layers of
 a) greater amentum
 b) lesser omentum
 c) falciform ligament
 d) ligamentum teres

1256. The ligamentum venosum is the fibrous remnant of
 a) left umbilical vein
 b) right umbilical vein
 c) ductus venosus
 d) ductus arteriosus

1257. The ligamentum venosum usually extends **between**
 a) left hepatic vein and left branch of portal vein
 b) left hepatic vein and right branch of portal vein
 c) right hepatic vein and right branch of portal vein
 d) right hepatic vein and left branch of portal vein

1258. Which of the following is the visceral surface of the liver?
 a) anterior b) posterior c) superior d) inferior

1259. Which of the following surfaces of liver present the fissure for ligamentum venosum?
 a) anterior b) posterior c) superior d) inferior

1260. Ligamentum teres of liver is the obliterated vestige of
 a) right umbilical artery
 b) left umbilical artery
 c) right umbilical vein
 d) left umbilical vein

1261. Ligamentum teres is attached to which of the following veins?
 a) right hepatic
 b) left hepatic
 c) left branch of portal
 d) right branch of portal

1262. All of the following structures lie at the porta hepatis **except**
 a) hepatic veins
 b) hepatic artery
 c) portal vein
 d) hepatic ducts

1263. The branches of portal vein and the tributaries of hepatic vein are more numerous
 a) before birth
 b) during childhood
 c) in young adults
 d) in old age

1264. The occasional projection from the lower border of the right lobe of liver to the right of gall bladder is known as
 a) Riedel's lobe
 b) caudate process
 c) quadrate lobe
 d) omental tuberosity

1265. All of the following vessels exist in relation to the liver **except**
 a) portal vein
 b) portal artery
 c) hepatic veins
 d) hepatic artery

1266. Free margin of lesser omentum contains all of the following structures **except**
 a) hepatic artery
 b) portal vein
 c) hepatic veins
 d) bile duct

1267. Which of the following structures form the central axis of the hepatic lobules?
 a) hepatic artery radicals
 b) bile duct radicals
 c) portal vein radicals
 d) central vein

Chapter VIII
Abdomen, Pelvis and Perineum 127

1268. In the sections of the liver a polygonal teritory centered on a portal triad, is termed as a
    a) hepatic lobule
    b) portal lobule
    c) portal acinus
    d) portal canal
1269. Which of the following is the most useful concept in considerations of the metabolic organization of the liver?
    a) hepatic lobule
    b) portal lobule
    c) portal acinus
    d) hepatic laminae
1270. Hepatocytes of liver are derived from which of following germ layers?
    a) ectoderm
    b) endoderm
    c) mesoderm
    d) all of the above
1271. Which of the following cells of the liver shows features indicating a high metabolic activity?
    a) hepatocytes
    b) cells of Kupffer
    c) endotheliocytes
    d) epitheliocytes
1272. Hepatocytes of which of the following zones of the hepatic lobule show features of highest metabolic activity?
    a) zone I
    b) zone II
    c) zone III
    d) all show equal metabolic activity
1273. In liver the stellate cells of Von Kupffer are present at which of the following sites?
    a) in the space of Moll
    b) in the perisinusoidal space
    c) on the luminal aspect of endotheliocytes of sinusoids
    d) on the abluminal aspect of the endothelial cells of sinusoids
1274. Which of the following is known as the 'space of Moll' in the liver?
    a) sinusoidal space
    b) perisinusoidal space
    c) perivascular space in portal canals
    d) lumen of the central vein
1275. The range of capacity of gall bladder is
    a) 30 - 50 ml
    b) 50 - 150 ml
    c) 150 - 300 ml
    d) 300 - 500 ml
1276. The gonadal ducts in the human female are derived from
    a) mesonephric ducts
    b) nephric tubules
    c) paramesonephric duct
    d) all of the above
1277. In human being the gonads develop from the
    a) ectoderm
    b) neural crest cells
    c) somites
    d) coelomic epithelium
1278. All of the following structures are related to the left kidney anteriorly except
    a) spleen
    b) stomach
    c) duodenum
    d) tail of pancreas

1279. All of the following areas on the anterior surface of right kidney are devoid of peritoneum **except**
 a) hepatic   b) suprarenal   c) duodenal   d) colic

1280. All of the following areas on the anterior surface of left kidney are covered with peritoneum **except**
 a) jejunal   b) splenic   c) gastric   d) pancreatic

1281. The usual relative position of the main hilar structures of kidney from before backwards is its
 a) artery, vein and pelvis
 b) pelvis, vein and artery
 c) vein, artery and pelvis
 d) vein, pelvis and artery

1282. Which of the following spaces is renal sinus?
 a) lumen of the renal pelvis
 b) central recess of the renal hilum
 c) site of opening of renal vein into inferior vena cava
 d) none of the above

1283. In all, in each kidney the number of minor calices is
 a) 2-3   b) 7-13   c) 14-23   d) 25-23

1284. Which of the following is known as the pararenal body?
 a) mass of adipose tissue in which kidney and its vessels are embedded.
 b) a sheath of fascia surrounding the kidney
 c) fat behind the renal fascia
 d) all of the above together

1285. Where in relation to the kidney is the perirenal fat thickest?
 a) along the borders
 b) at the poles
 c) along the posterior surface
 d) along the anterior surface

1286. The anterior and posterior layers of renal fascia does not fuse
 a) surperiorly
 b) inferiorly
 c) medially
 d) laterally

1287. Part of renal cortex between the pyramids is known as
 a) pyramid
 b) cortical lobule
 c) renal column
 d) lobe of kidney

1288. Which of the following forms the lobe of the kidney?
 a) a renal pyramid plus the cortical cap covering it
 b) two renal pyramids plus intervening renal column
 c) two renal columns plus intervening pyramid
 d) two renal columns plus the joining peripheral cortex

1289. Which of the following parts of the uriniferous tubules of the kidney is concerned with selective absorption of the substances from the glomerular filtrate?
 a) renal corpuscle
 b) renal tubule
 c) collecting tubule
 d) all of the above

1290. All of the following statements pertaining to the glomerulus of kidney are correct **except** that
   a) it is a lobulated tuft of capillaries
   b) it is a enveloped by small pouch like commencement of a renal tubule
   c) its afferent vessel is an arteriole
   d) its efferent vessel is a venule

1291. Which of the following cells of the renal corpuscle are phagocytic in nature?
   a) podocytes
   b) endothelial cells
   c) mesangial cells
   d) cells lining parietal layer of Bowman's capsule

1292. Which of the following part of the loop of Henle is known as a thick segment?
   a) upper part of ascending limb
   b) lower part of ascending limb
   c) upper part of descending limb
   d) lower part of descending limb

1293. The special thickened region, macula densa of the renal tubule lies between the
   a) loop of Henle and distal convoluted tubule
   b) straight and convoluted portions of distal convoluted tubule
   c) distal convoluted tubule and junctional tubule
   d) junctional tubule and connecting duct

1294. Cells lining which of the following part of the renal tubule bear tall microvilli?
   a) proximal convoluted tubule
   b) neck
   c) loop of Henle
   d) distal convoluted tubule

1295. Which of the following are juxtaglomerular cells in the juxtaglomerular apparatus of kidney?
   a) podocytes
   b) mesangial cells
   c) smooth cells of afferent and efferent arterioles
   d) modified lining cells of distal convoluted tubule

1296. Modified columnar cells of distal convoluted tubule at juxtaglomerular apparatus are known as
   a) mesangial cells
   b) podocytes
   c) juxtaglomerular cells
   d) macula densa cells

1297. All of the following constitute juxtaglomerular apparatus **except**
   a) podocytes
   b) mesangeal element
   c) juxtaglomercular cells
   d) macula densa

1298. Accessory renal arteries when present usually arise from
   a) coeliac artery
   b) superior mesenteric artery
   c) aorta
   d) common iliac artery

1299. Which of the following places is the narrowest region of ureter?
    a) its mid point
    b) at its junction with renal pelvis
    c) at the point where it crosses the pelvic brim
    d) as it passess through the wall of urinary bladder

1300. The right ureter is crossed from front by all of the following vessels **except**
    a) ileocolic
    b) inferior mesentric
    c) right colic
    d) right gonadal

1301. The epithelium of ureter is the
    a) stratified squamous
    b) psueudostratified columnar
    c) transitional
    d) simple columnar

1302. In adults, the filling of the urinary bladder may be permitted upto about
    a) 200 ml
    b) 300 ml
    c) 500 ml
    d) 1000 ml

1303. The needle pierces all of the following structures in order to drain the hydrocele of testes, **except**
    a) tunica albugenia
    b) tunica vaginalis
    c) internal spermatic fascia
    d) cremasteric fascia

1304. The slit of male urethral canal is transversely arched in which of the following parts?
    a) prostatic
    b) membranous
    c) spongiose
    d) at the external orific

1305. Which of the following male structures is thought to be the homologue of the female vagina?
    a) prostate
    b) prostatic utricle
    c) prostatic sinus
    d) navicular fossa of urethra

1306. Which of the following parts of the male urethra is lined by the transitional epithelium?
    a) near the external urethral orifice
    b) spongy
    c) prostatic
    d) membranous

1307. A cyst found in association with the head of the epididymis is known as
    a) infantile hydrocele
    b) paradidymis
    c) spermatocele
    d) encysted hydrocele of the cord

1308. The artery of the ductus deference is usually derived from which of the following artery?
    a) superior vesicle
    b) aorta
    c) internal iliac
    d) common iliac

Chapter VIII — Abdomen, Pelvis and Perineum

1309. During which of the following periods of life, the endometrium lining the body of the uterus undergoes monthly cyclical changes?
   a) throughout the whole life
   b) before puberty
   c) after menopause
   d) between puberty and menopause

1310. Which of the following structures is suspended by numerous suspensory ligaments?
   a) thyroid gland
   b) mammary gland
   c) ileo-jejunal flexure
   d) penis

1311. A condition in which there is occassional hypertrophy of the male mammary gland after puberty is known as
   a) amastia
   b) gynaecomastia
   c) polymastia
   d) athelia

1312. Notch on the inferior border of liver for ligamentum teres is
   a) in the midline
   b) to the right of midline
   c) to the left of midline
   d) variable in relation to midline

1313. Which part of the inferior border of liver is accessible to percussion in adults?
   a) whole of it
   b) below the right costal margin
   c) below the left costal margin
   d) at the infrasternal angle

1314. All of the following superficial features of liver form the original basis for demarcation of right and left lobes **except**
   a) attachment of falciform fold
   b) fissure for inferior vena cava
   c) fissure for ligamentus teres
   d) fissure for ligamentum venosum

1315. What is the position of the dividing zone between the right and left functional lobes of liver in relation to its traditional surface demarcation?
   a) overlapping
   b) right
   c) right
   d) variable

1316. Quadrate lobe of liver is bounded by all of the following **except**
   a) fissure for ligamentum teres
   b) porta hepatis
   c) fossa for gall bladder
   d) fissure for inferior vena cava

1317. Caudate lobe of liver is bounded on the left by
   a) fissure for ligamentum teres
   b) fissure for inferior vena cava
   c) fissure for ligamentum venosum
   d) fossa for gall bladder

1318. All of the following structures are connected directly to the liver by peritoneum **except**
   a) stomach
   b) duodenum
   c) transverse colon
   d) diaphragm

1319. Which of the following structures related to liver is not a fold of peritoneum?
　　a) lesser omentum　　b) ligamentum teres
　　c) falciform ligament　　d) coronary ligaments
1320. Which of the following gives attachment to the lower end of ligamentum venosum?
　　a) left hepatic vein　　b) right hepatic vein
　　c) hepatic artery　　d) left branch of portal vein
1321. Upper end of ligamentum venosum is attached to
　　a) right hepatic vein　　b) left hepatic vein
　　c) hepatic artery　　d) portal vein
1322. Part of caudate lobe at the summit of the fissure for ligamentum venosum and the porta hepatis is called as
　　a) caudate process　　b) papillary process
　　c) omental tuberosity　　d) Riedel's lobe
1323. The ligamentum teres is attached at its upper end to
　　a) left branch of portal vein　　b) right branch of portal vein
　　c) left hepatic vein　　d) right hepatic vein
1324. When the inferior border of liver to the right of gall bladder projects down as a linguiform process it is known as
　　a) omental tuberosity　　b) Riedel's lobe
　　c) caudate process　　d) fibrous appendix of liver
1325. At the left end of the liver in adults a fibrous band when present is known as
　　a) papillary process　　b) Riedel's lobe
　　c) appendix of liver　　d) coronary ligament
1326. Atrophied remnants of more extensive left lobe of liver of early life is represented in adults by
　　a) Riedel's lobe　　b) appendix of liver
　　c) papillary process　　d) omental tuberosity

Chapter IX

HEAD, FACE, NECK AND NERVOUS SYSTEM

1327. In adults, the lower end of spinal cord corresponds with the lower border of
    a) first coccygeal segment
    b) last coccygeal segment
    c) first sacral segment
    d) first lumbar vertebra

1328. Average length of the adult spinal cord is
    a) 25 cm
    b) 40 cm
    c) 45 cm
    d) 60 cm

1329. Lower end of filum terminale is attached to the dorsum of
    a) first lumbar vertebra
    b) last lumbar vertebra
    c) last sacral segment
    d) first coccygeal segment

1330. Which spinal segment of cervical enlargement of spinal cord shows maximum circumference?
    a) fourth
    b) fifth
    c) sixth
    d) seventh

1331. Which of the following vertebral levels correspond with the lumbar enlargement of the spinal cord?
    a) seventh to tenth thoracic
    b) ninth to twelfth thoracic
    c) eleventh thoracic to first lumbar
    d) tenth thoracic to first lumbar

1332. Extension of dural and arachnoid meninges surround the filum terminale in its
    a) upper 5 cm
    b) upper 10 cm
    c) upper 15 cm
    d) whole length

1333. Dura and arachnoid meninges extend upto the lower border of which of the following vertebra?
    a) first lumbar
    b) second lumbar
    c) second sacral
    d) first coccygeal

1334. The central canal is continued in the filum terminale for
    a) 0.06 mm
    b) 0.56 mm
    c) 5.6 mm
    d) 56 mm

1335. The site of election for spinal puncture is
    a) subarachnoid space around the filum terminale internum
    b) subdural space around the filum terminale internum
    c) central canal contained in the filum terminale internum
    d) central canal contained in conus medullaris

1336. Ventral and dorsal roots of spinal nerves meet
   a) outside the intervertebral foramina
   b) in the intervertebral foramina
   c) in the subdural space
   d) in the subarachnoid space

1337. Which of the following defines the 'cauda equina'?
   a) the fibrous filament extending from the lower end of spinal cord
   b) the lower conical part of spinal cord
   c) the bunch of nerves around the filum terminale
   d) the lumbar spinal enlargement

1338. Regarding the central and peripheral processes of the spinal ganglia neuron which of the following statements is correct?
   a) both are the axons
   b) both are the dendrites
   c) central process is an axon and the peripheral one a dendrite
   d) central process is a dendrite and the peripheral one an axon

1339. The 'spinal segment' can be defined as the part of the spinal cord giving rise to
   a) one spinal nerve
   b) one spinal rootlet
   c) a pair of spinal rootlets
   d) a pair of spinal nerves

1340. All of the following cells are seen in the spinal cord **except**
   a) oligodendrocytes
   b) microglia
   c) neurons
   d) Schwann cells

1341. The lateral (horn) gray column of the spinal cord is confined to the segments between
   a) first cervical to first coccygeal
   b) third cervical to first thoracic
   c) ninth thoracic to third lumbar.
   d) second thoracic to first lumbar

1342. In the cervical spinal cord the reticular formation is seen in the region of
   a) outer aspect of funiculi
   b) between dorsal funiculi and posterior commissure
   c) between lateral funiculi and gray matter
   d) between anterior funiculi and anterior commissure

1343. Which region of the spinal cord shows gray matter absolutely and relatively small in volume?
   a) cervical
   b) thoracic
   c) lumbar
   d) sacral

1344. Terminal ventricle represents the vertricular system of nervous system in
   a) cerebrum
   b) diencephalon
   c) midbrain
   d) conus medullaris

1345. Posterior median septum is thickest in which region of the spinal cord?
    a) cervical
    b) thoracic
    c) sacral
    d) lumbar
1346. The so-called gray appearance of the spinal gray matter is due to the predominance of
    a) neuronal somata
    b) neurites
    c) neuroglia
    d) blood vessels
1347. Neurons with their axons passing out of the gray matter in the ventral spinal roots or spinal tracts are knows as
    a) Golgi type - I
    b) Golgi type - II
    c) intersegmental
    d) intrasegmental
1348. Nucleus dorsalis can be usually identified in the spinal cord segments
    a) eighth cervical to third lumbar
    b) second cervical to first lumbar
    c) third cervical to first thoracic
    d) ninth thoracic to first lumbar
1349. Parasympathetic gray column is confined to spinal cord segments
    a) third cervical to first thoracic
    b) second cervical to first lumbar
    c) ninth thoracic to first thoracic
    d) second to fourth sacral
1350. Fibres from neurons of all of the following form the longitudinal spinal tracts **except**
    a) dorsal root ganglia
    b) sensory neurons in the dorsal gray column
    c) motor neurons in the ventral gray column
    d) intra- and intersegmental neurons
1351. Which of the following is the descending spinal tract?
    a) fasciculus gracilis
    b) dorsolateral
    c) pyramidal (corticospinal)
    d) fasciculus cuneatus
1352. In which funiculus of the spinal cord is the vestibulospinal tract located?
    a) anterior
    b) lateral
    c) posterior
    d) lateral and posterior
1353. All of the following tracts are located in the anterior funiculus of the spinal cord **except**
    a) vestibulospinal
    b) tectospinal
    c) rubrospinal
    d) reticulospinal
1354. All of the following tracts are predominantly un-crossed **except**
    a) reticulospinal
    b) vestibulospinal
    c) tectospinal
    d) interstitiospinal

1355. Which of the following tracts descends in the anterior funiculus of the whole spinal cord?
   a) reticulospinal
   b) tectospinal
   c) vestibulospinal
   d) anterior corticospinal

1356. Which of the following tracts is said to be concerned with crude tactile and pressure sensibility?
   a) fasciculus gracilis
   b) anterior spinothalamic
   c) lateral spinothalamic
   d) fasciculus cuneatus

1357. Of the total fibres contained in the lateral corticospinal tract myelinated are nearly
   a) 20%
   b) 50%
   c) 70%
   d) 100%

1358. Majority of the fibres of the pyramidal pathway originate from Brodmann's cortical area
   a) 3, 1, 2
   b) 4
   c) 6
   d) 17

1359. In the tracts of the spinal cord longer fibres are said to be placed
   a) superficially
   b) deeply
   c) intermediate
   d) randomly

1360. Most corticospinal fibres probably synapse with
   a) anterior horn neurons directly
   b) posterior horn neurons
   c) interneurons in the base of dorsal gray columns
   d) interneurons in the anterior gray column

1361. Which of the following tracts passes through the inferior cerebellar peduncle?
   a) tractus gracilis
   b) posterior spinocerebellar
   c) anterior spinocerebellar
   d) spinotectal

1362. Fibres arising from the ipsilateral thoracic nucleus gives rise to
   a) anterior spinocerebellar tract
   b) posterior spinocerebellar tract
   c) lateral spinothalamic
   d) fasciculus gracilis

1363. In which funiculus of the spinal cord is anterior spinocerebellar tract located?
   a) anterior
   b) lateral
   c) posterior
   d) lateral and posterior

1364. Exteroceptive and proprioceptive impulses from the trunk and lower limb are chiefly carried by
   a) anterior spinocerebellar tract
   b) posterior spinocerebellar tract
   c) anterior spinothalamic tract
   d) gracilis fasciculus

Chapter IX   Head, Face, Neck and Nervous System   **137**

1365. Tract carrying the proprioceptive impulses from the upper limbs is
   a) tractus gracilis   b) posterior spinocerebellar
   c) anterior spinocerebellar   d) cuneocerebellar
1366. Which of the following tract is the major path serving somatic pain and thermal sensibilities?
   a) lateral spinothalamic   b) anterior spinothalamic
   c) fasciculus gracilis   d) fasciculus cuneatus
1367. Which of the following tracts provides the route for the spinovisual reflexes?
   a) spinorubral   b) spinoreticular
   c) spinothalamic   d) spinotectal
1368. Which of the following tracts carries the impulses evoking the movement of the head and eyes towards the source of stimulation?
   a) cuneocerebellar   b) spinotectal
   c) spinothalamic   d) spinorubral
1369. Which of the following tracts is situated between the apex of the posterior gray column and the surface of spinal cord?
   a) dorsolateral   b) spinoreticular
   c) spinoolivary   d) spinotectal
1370. Which of the following fibres intermingle with fibres of spinothalamic tract in the spinal cord?
   a) spinoolivary   b) spinotectal
   c) spinoreticular   d) spinocerebellar
1371. All of the following statements regarding fasciculus cuneatus are correct **except**
   a) it commences at midthoracic level of spinal cord
   b) it is medial to fasciculus gracilis
   c) some of its axons are secondary from ipsilateral dorsal gray column
   d) its fibres are larger than those of fasciculus gracilis
1372. Which of the following statements regarding fasciculus gracilis is correct?
   a) It contains the ascending branches of axons of spinal ganglia.
   b) It commences at midthoracic spinal level.
   c) It is lateral to fasciculus cuneatus.
   d) Lower fibres are pushed laterally by successive addition.
1373. Which of the following tracts mainly contains primary afferent neurons?
   a) tractus gracilis and cuneatus   b) spinothalamic
   c) anterior spinocerebellar   d) posterior spinocerebellar
1374. Afferent neurons in gracile and cuneate nuclei are mainly
   a) primary   b) secondary
   c) tertiary   d) all type

1375. Which of the following belongs to the proprioceptive pathway?
   a) medial lemniscus
   b) internal arcuate fibres
   c) posterior external arcuate fibres
   d) all of above
1376. Which of the following thalamic nuclei receives the fibres of medial lemniscus?
   a) ventral
   b) medial
   c) ventroposteromedial (VPM)
   d) ventroposterolateral (VPL)
1377. Lesions of spinal cord at C5 spinal segment will result in
   a) respiratory failure
   b) quadriplegia
   c) hemiplegia
   d) paraplegia
1378. Which spinal segment is in level with the spine of twelfth thoracic vertebra in adult?
   a) twelfth thoracic
   b) first lumbar
   c) second lumbar
   d) first sacral
1379. The neonatal spinal cord extends to the upper border of which vertebra?
   a) first lumbar
   b) third lumbar
   c) second sacral
   d) third sacral
1380. Telencephalon of developing brain gives rise to
   a) pons and cerebellum
   b) medulla oblongata
   c) cerebrum
   d) cerebrum amd thalamus
1381. Masses of somata of neurons in the central nervous system are called as
   a) ganglia
   b) tracts
   c) nuclei
   d) peduncles
1382. Pons is derived from
   a) telecephalon
   b) metencephalon
   c) myelencephalon
   d) mesencephalon
1383. All of the following statements regarding the medulla oblongata are correct **except**
   a) it is derived from myelencephalon
   b) its lower extent corresponds with the centre of dens ventrally
   c) its lower half forms half the floor of fourth ventricle
   d) its closed part contains the central canal
1384. Fascicles of pyramidal decussation can be seen crossing obliquely on surface of
   a) basillar sulcus
   b) anterior median fissure of spinal cord
   c) anterior median fissure of medulla oblongata
   d) interpeducular sulcus

Head, Face, Neck and Nervous System

385. Rootlets of which of the following nerves are in line with the ventral spinal roots?
    a) facial
    b) glossopharyngeal
    c) accessory
    d) hypoglossal

386. Rootlets of all of the following nerves are in line with the dorsal spinal roots **except**
    a) abducent
    b) accessory
    c) glossopharyngeal
    d) vagus

387. Rootlets of hypoglossal nerve emerge through which of the sulcus/fissure of medulla oblongata?
    a) anterior median fissure
    b) posterior median fissure
    c) anterolateral sulcus
    d) posterolateral sulcus

388. All of the following nerves are attached at the pontomedullary junction **except**
    a) trigeminal
    b) abducent
    c) facial
    d) vestibulocochlear

389. What percentage of the fibres of corticospinal pathway cross in the pyramidal decussation?
    a) 100%
    b) 10-30%
    c) 70-90%
    d) 50%

390. Fibres that cross the olive externally are
    a) internal arcuate
    b) anterior external arcuate
    c) stria medullaris
    d) post-external arcuate

391. Sometimes on the surface of medulla oblongata tuberculum cinerium can be seen in between
    a) gracile and cuneate tubercles
    b) gracile tubercle and posterior median sulcus
    c) cuneate fasciculus and rootlets of accessory nerve
    d) pyramid and olive

392. Substantia gelatinosa of spinal cord continues in the medulla oblongata as
    a) nucleus of spinal tract of trigeminal
    b) accessory nucleus
    c) gracile nucleus
    d) cuneate nucleus

393. Which of the following is formed from the axons of the nuclei gracilis and cuneatus?
    a) fasciculi gracilis and cuneatus
    b) stria medullaris
    c) internal arcuate fibres
    d) anterior external arcuate fibres

394. Which of the following lemniscus contains secondary neuron fibres in the proprioceptive pathway?
    a) spinal
    b) medial
    c) lateral
    d) all of the above

1395. Posterior external arcuate fibres originate from
    a) arcuate nuclei
    b) nucleus gracilis
    c) nucleus cuneatus
    d) accessory cuneate nucleus

1396. Cuneocerebellar tract carries proprioceptive impulses from
    a) head
    b) thorax
    c) upper limb
    d) whole body

1397. The nucleus of the spinal tract of trigeminal nerve is separated from the surface of the cord by
    a) internal arcuate fibres
    b) spinal tract of trigeminal
    c) inferior cerebellar peduncle
    d) dorsal spinocerebellar tract

1398. All vagal visceral afferent neurons terminate in
    a) nucleus solitarius
    b) nucleus ambiguus
    c) dorsal vagal nucleus
    d) nucleus intercalatus

1399. The tractus solitarius receives afferents from all of the following nerves except
    a) facial
    b) glossopharyngeal
    c) vagus
    d) trigeminal

1400. Coordination of movements of eyes and head in response to vestibulocochlear stimulation is the chief function of
    a) vestibulospinal tract
    b) lateral lemniscus
    c) tectospinal tract
    d) medial longitudinal fasciculus

1401. All of the statements regarding the inferior olivary nucleus are correct except
    a) it lies dorsolateral to the pyramids
    b) it is irregularly crenated
    c) the olivocerebellar fibres enter the ipsilateral inferior cerebellar peduncle
    d) ascending afferent fibres to it are mainly crossed

1402. Which of the following nuclei are said to be the displaced pontine nuclei
    a) accessory olivary nuclei
    b) arcuate nuclei
    c) salivatory nuclei
    d) all of the above

1403. Fibres originating from arcuate nuclei give rise to
    a) internal arcuate fibres
    b) anterior external arcuate fibres
    c) posterior external arcuate fibres
    d) middle cerebellar peduncle

1404. Fibres arising from nucleus ambiguous join all of the following nerves except
    a) glossopharyngeal
    b) vagus
    c) accessory
    d) hypoglossal

Head, Face, Neck and Nervous System 141

405. Which of the following nuclei lies superficial to the inferior cerebellar peduncle?
    a) auditory
    b) vestibular
    c) vagal
    d) spinal nucleus of trigeminal

406. Stria medullaris of fourth ventricle are
    a) cuneocerebellar fibres
    b) auditory nerve fibres
    c) aberrant pontocerebellar fibres
    d) vestibulocerebellar fibres

407. The spinal lemniscus contains the fibres from
    a) nuclei gracilis and cuneatus
    b) auditory nuclei
    c) nuclei of trigeminal nerves
    d) spinothalamic tract

408. Which of the following peduncles connects pons with the cerebellum?
    a) cerebral
    b) superior cerebellar
    c) middle cerebellar
    d) inferior cerebellar

409. Sulcus basillaris is present on ventral surface of
    a) midbrain
    b) pons
    c) medulla oblongata
    d) cerebellum

410. Which of the following nerves delimits pons from middle cerebellar peduncle?
    a) oculomotor
    b) trochlear
    c) trigeminal
    d) facial

411. The tegmentum of pons is the continuation of medulla oblongata excluding its
    a) pyramids
    b) olive
    c) ascending tracts
    d) nuclei

412. The pathway formed by nuclei pontis is
    a) corticopontospinal
    b) corticopontocerebellar
    c) corticopontonuclear
    d) corticopontothalamic

413. All of the following fibres are contained in the ventral (basillar) part of pons **except**
    a) corticospinal
    b) corticopontine
    c) pontocerebellar
    d) medial lemniscus

414. All of the following nuclei are present in the tegmentum of pons **except**
    a) nuclei pontis
    b) abducent nerve nucelus
    c) facial nerve nucleus
    d) vestibular nuclei

415. The vestibular group of nuclei sends fibres to all of the following **except**
    a) cerebellum
    b) medial longitudinal fasciculus
    c) spinal cord
    d) medial lemniscus

416. Nerve fibres entering the medulla oblongata between the inferior cerebellar peduncle and the spinal trigeminal tract are from
    a) trigeminal nerve
    b) facial nerve
    c) vestibular part of vestibulocochlear nerve
    d) auditory part of vestibulocochlear nerve

1417. Which of the following nuclei is present at the pontomedullar junction?
   a) abducent
   b) facial
   c) auditory
   d) vagal

1418. Fibres of trapezoid body of pons originate from
   a) cerebral cortex
   b) inferior colliculus
   c) auditory nuclei
   d) cerebellar cortex

1419. All of the following belong to the auditory pathway **except**
   a) superior olivary nucleus
   b) trapezoid body
   c) lateral lemniscus
   d) vestibular nuclei

1420. Which of the following lemniscus carries the fibres of auditor pathway?
   a) lateral
   b) medial
   c) spinal
   d) trigeminal

1421. Which of the following are involved in the aberrant corticoponto cerebellar connection?
   a) arcuate nuclei
   b) stria medullaris of fourth ventricle
   c) anterior external arcuate fibres
   d) all of the above

1422. All of the following nuclei form a somatic motor column **except**
   a) trochlear
   b) oculomotor
   c) hypoglossal
   d) facial

1423. Facial colliculus in the floor of rhomboid fossa is caused due underlying
   a) facial nucleus
   b) abducent nucleus
   c) auditory nucleus
   d) vestibular nuclei

1424. The course of fibres from which of the following nucleus provide an apparent evidence for neurobiotaxis
   a) facial
   b) abducent
   c) trochlear
   d) auditory

1425. The facial nucleus connects fibres from all of the following **except**
   a) cerebral cortex
   b) cerebellar cortex
   c) nucleus solitarius
   d) spinal trigeminal nucleus

1426. Facial nucleus neurons which are believed to receive bilater corticonuclear fibres innervate muscles in the
   a) scalp only
   b) scalp and upper face only
   c) lower face only
   d) whole face

1427. Trapezoid body of pons is formed by decussation of fibres from
   a) gracile and cuneate nuclei
   b) auditory nuclei
   c) trigeminal nerve nuclei
   d) nuclei pontis

1428. All of the following nuclei form the relay stations in the **acoustic** pathway **except**
   a) superior olivary nuclei
   b) inferior olivary nuclei
   c) trapezoid nuclei
   d) nuclei of lateral lemniscus

1429. Which of the following nuclei sends secretomotor fibres to the **lacrimal** gland?
   a) accessory oculomotor
   b) superior salivary
   c) inferior salivary
   d) nucleus ambiguus

1430. The spinal tract of trigeminal consists of axons from
   a) main sensory nucleus of trigeminal
   b) dorsal horn of spinal cord
   c) trigeminal ganglia
   d) spinal nucleus of trigeminal

1431. The trigeminal lemniscus consists of fibres from
   a) trigeminal ganglia
   b) dorsal horn of spinal cord
   c) ventroposteromedial nucleus of thalamus
   d) spinal and principal nucleus of trigeminal

1432. In the tegmentum, the arrangement of the lemnisci in lateral order from midline is
   a) medial, lateral, spinal, trigeminal
   b) medial, spinal, lateral, trigeminal
   c) medial, spinal, trigeminal, lateral
   d) medial, trigeminal, spinal, lateral

1433. Which of the following lemniscus forms the ascending auditory path?
   a) medial
   b) lateral
   c) trigeminal
   d) spinal

1434. The main 'intersegmental tract' in the brain stem is
   a) medial longitudinal fasciculus
   b) cerebral peduncle
   c) dorsal tegmental fascical
   d) medial lemniscus

1435. Secondary axons from the principle trigeminal sensory nucleus ascend to thalamus in the
   a) trigeminal lemniscus
   b) spinal lemniscus
   c) medial lemniscus
   d) medial longitudinal fasciculus

1436. Which of the following lemnisci terminates in the inferior colliculus?
   a) medial
   b) lateral
   c) spinal
   d) trigeminal

1437. Which of the following fibres are contained in the superior cerebellar peduncle?
   a) dentatorubral
   b) pontocerebellar
   c) olivocerebellar
   d) vestibulocerebellar

1438. In adults the ratio of cerebellum to cerebrum is
   a) 1 to 4
   b) 1 to 8
   c) 1 to 16
   d) 1 to 20

1439. Vallecula of the cerebellum separates
   a) its upper and lower halves ventrally
   b) its upper and lower halves dorsally
   c) right and left hemispheres superiosly
   d) right and left hemispheres inferiorly

1440. All of the following statements regarding fissura prima of cerebellum are correct **except**
   a) it is the deepest fissure on the superior surface
   b) it is somewhat V-shaped
   c) it cuts the superior vermis into anterior 1/3 and posterior 2/3
   d) it separates the anterior lobe from middle lobe

1441. Which of the following part of the vermis of cerebellum is continuous with the superior medullary vellum?
   a) central lobule
   b) uvula
   c) lingula
   d) nodule

1442. All of the following parts of the vermis are continuos bilaterally with an adjoining lobule **except**
   a) uvula
   b) lingula
   c) central lobule
   d) culmen

1443. Which of the following parts of the cerebellar vermis are seperated by the dorsolateral fissure from each other?
   a) uvula and nodule
   b) uvula and pyramid
   c) nodule and lingula
   d) tuber and pyramid

1444. Phylongetically oldest part of the cerebellum is
   a) floculonodular lobe
   b) only the vermis
   c) corpus cerebelli
   d) anterior lobe

1445. Cerebellum develops from
   a) myelencephalon
   b) metencephalon
   c) telencephalon
   d) diencephalon

1446. All of the following parts of the vermis belong to neocerebellum **except**
   a) central lobule
   b) culmen
   c) pyramid
   d) tuber

1447. Which of the following parts of vermis belongs to the neocerebellum?
   a) nodule
   b) tuber
   c) lingula
   d) uvula

1448. All of the following parts of cerebellum belong to the archicerebellum **except**
   a) flocculus
   b) lingula
   c) tonsil
   d) nodule

1449. Which of the following parts of the anterior lobe of cerebellum belongs to archicerebellum?
   a) lingula
   b) central lobule
   c) ala
   d) culmen

Chapter IX Head, Face, Neck and Nervous System

450. Middle cerebellar peduncle of the cerebellum connects the cerebellum with
   a) midbrain
   b) pons
   c) medulla oblongata
   d) spinal cord
451. Juxtarestiform body is the part of which of the following peduncles?
   a) cerebral
   b) superior cerebellar
   c) middle cerebellar
   d) inferior cerebellar
452. All of the following tracts enter the cerebellum through inferior cerebellar peduncle **except**
   a) ventral spinocerebellar
   b) vestibulocerebellar
   c) olivocerebellar
   d) dorsal spino-cerebellar
453. All of the following fibres/tracts/peduncles belong to the corticoponto-cerebellar pathway **except**
   a) middle cerebellar peduncle
   b) ventral external arcuate fibres
   c) stria medullaris
   d) internal arcuate fibres
454. All of the following tracts pass to cerebellum through superior cerebellar peduncle **except**
   a) superior spinocerebellar
   b) ventral spinocerebellar
   c) dorsal spinocerebellar
   d) tectocerebellar
455. Which of the following is represented by spinocerebellum?
   a) neocerebellum
   b) archicerebellum
   c) paleocerebellum
   d) all of the above
456. All of the following are intracerebellar nuclei **except**
   a) ambiguus
   b) dentate
   c) fastigial
   d) globose
457. Axons from which of the following neurons synapse with the neurons of intracerebellar nuclei?
   a) Golgi
   b) basket
   c) stellate
   d) Purkinje
458. The only axons leaving the cerebellar cortex originate from which of the following neuron?
   a) Purkinje
   b) Golgi
   c) granular
   d) basket
459. Disturbances in the muscular integration is the most obvious effect of dysfunction of
   a) cerebral cortex motor area
   b) thalamus
   c) hypothalamus
   d) cerebellar cortex
460. Mossy afferents to cerebellar cortex originate from all of the following **except**
   a) dorsal column of spinal cord
   b) inferior olivary nucleus
   c) vestibular nuclei
   d) reticular formation

1461. Climbing fibres to the cerebellar cortex originate from
   a) dorsal thoracic nucleus
   b) vestibular nuclei
   c) reticular formation
   d) inferior olivary nucleus

1462. Which of the following afferents exert a one-to-one, all or none excitation on the individual Purkinje neuron?
   a) climbing fibres
   b) mossy fibres
   c) both a & b
   d) none of the above

1463. A defect in the rapid alternating movements is known as
   a) asynergia
   b) dysequillibrium
   c) ataxia
   d) dysdiadochokinesis

1464. All of the following are the effects of cerebellar dysfunction **except**
   a) astereognosis
   b) ataxia
   c) asthenia
   d) asynergia

1465. The dorsal layer of tela choroidea of the fourth ventricle covers
   a) inferior vermis
   b) inferior surface of cerebellar hemispheres
   c) roof of fourth ventricle
   d) floor of fourth ventricle

1466. Apertures in the wall of which ventricle drain the CSF from ventricular system to the subarachnoid space?
   a) lateral
   b) third
   c) fourth
   d) all of the above

1467. Which ventricles are communicated by the interventricular foramina?
   a) third and fourth
   b) lateral and third
   c) lateral and fourth
   d) right and left lateral

1468. Tela choroidea can be defined as
   a) a double fold of pia mater
   b) vascular fringes in the pial fold
   c) double fold of ependyma with vascular fringes
   d) single layer of pia matter with the ependyma

1469. Which of the following artery forms the choroid plexus of fourth ventricle?
   a) middle cerebral
   b) posterior cerebral
   c) inferior cerebellar
   d) superior cerebellar

1470. Inferior apex of the floor of fourth ventricle is known as
   a) obex
   b) calamus scriptorius
   c) area postrema
   d) finiculus

1471. Which of the following defines the cerebral peduncle?
   a) each half of midbrain
   b) crus cerebri with substantia nigra
   c) part of midbrain behind substantia nigra
   d) each half of midbrain in front of transverse line passing through cerebral aqueduct

Chapter IX Head, Face, Neck and Nervous System 147

1472. Whole part of midbrain behind the crura cerebri is known as
    a) tectum
    b) tegmentum
    c) substantia nigra
    d) cerebral peduncle
1473. Fibres contained in crura cerebri are
    a) corticospinal
    b) corticopontine
    c) corticonuclear
    d) all of the above
1474. Nerve roots emerging from the medial sulcus of crus cerebri are of
    a) oculomotor
    b) trigeminal
    c) trochlear
    d) optic
1475. Which of the following cranial nerves crosses the lateral surface of cerebral peuduncle?
    a) optic
    b) oculomotor
    c) olfactory
    d) trochlear
1476. Which of the following forms a relay station for visual pathway?
    a) thalamus
    b) pineal body
    c) superior colliculus
    d) inferior colliculus
1477. All of the following statements regarding the brachium of superior colliculus are correct **except**
    a) it overlaps the medial geniculate body
    b) it continues into the lateral geniculate body
    c) it is involved in visual pathway
    d) it conveys fibres from lateral lemniscus
1478. Neurons of which of the following nucleus contain ferric pigment?
    a) mesencephalic
    b) Edinger-Westphal
    c) red
    d) subthalamic
1479. Which of the following is the cavity of diencephalon?
    a) lateral ventricle
    b) third ventricle
    c) fourth ventricle
    d) cerebral aqueduct
1480. All of the following constitute the epithalamus **except**
    a) habenular nuclei
    b) posterior commissure
    c) geniculate bodies
    d) epiphysis cerebri
1481. The anterior limit of the median part of the forebrain is represented by
    a) stria terminalis
    b) stria medullaris
    c) lamina terminalis
    d) corpus callosum
1482. Anterior boundary of interventricular foramen of brain is formed by
    a) anterior pole of thalamus
    b) fornix
    c) anterior commissure
    d) lamina terminalis

1483. All of the following statements regarding the interthalamic adhesion are correct **except**
   a) it connects two thalami
   b) it lies in front of interventricular foramen
   c) it contains neurons
   d) sometimes it is absent

1484. Which of the following parts of thalamus is neothalamus?
   a) anterior
   b) lateral
   c) medial
   d) anterior and medial

1485. Which of the following thalamic peduncles connects the **medial** geniculate body with the temporal cortex?
   a) frontal
   b) dorsal
   c) posterior
   d) ventral

1486. Thalamic nuclei which have multiple subcortical connections are known as
   a) relay nuclei
   b) association nuclei
   c) cortically dependent nuclei
   d) specific nuclei

1487. Which of the following thalamic nuclei receives the fibres of medial lemniscus?
   a) ventroposterolateral
   b) ventroposteromedial
   c) ventralis anterior
   d) ventralis intermedius

1488. Which of the following thalamic nuclear groups receives the mammilothalamic tract?
   a) pulvinar
   b) anterior group
   c) medial group
   d) lateral group

1489. The thalamocortical fibres from the anterior thalamic nucleus pass to
   a) limbic cortex
   b) visual cortex
   c) auditory cortex
   d) primary somatic sensory cortex

1490. The effects of ablation of which thalamic nuclei partly parallel with the results of prefrontal lobecotomy?
   a) medial group
   b) lateral group
   c) anterior group
   d) pulvinar

1491. Which of the following is the function of medial group of thalamic nuclei?
   a) recent memory
   b) integration of diverse sensory channels
   c) link in ascending activating system
   d) equillibrium

1492. Which of the following thalamic nucleus receives the fibres of gustatory pathway?
   a) ventralis anterior
   b) ventralis intermedius
   c) ventroposterolateral (VPL)
   d) ventroposteromedial (VPM)

Chapter IX   Head, Face, Neck and Nervous System   149

1493. Thalmus is involved in activities of the whole sensory system **except**
    a) gustatory
    b) visual
    c) auditory
    d) olfactory
1494. The thalamus is essential for the perception of all the sensory modalities **except**
    a) visual
    b) gustatory
    c) olfactory
    d) auditory
1495. The habenular nucleus is a station on the reflex route of
    a) vision
    b) olfaction
    c) taste
    d) audition
1496. Discrete lesions of one subthalamic nucleus result in
    a) tremors
    b) hemiballismus
    c) disequillibrium
    d) hemiplegia
1497. All of the following are in the lateral relation of the hypothalamus **except**
    a) lamina terminalis
    b) optic tract
    c) internal capsule
    d) anterior part of subthalamus
1498. 'Herring bodies' are seen in
    a) pineal gland
    b) neurohypophysis
    c) adenohypophysis
    d) hypothalamus
1499. Which of the following structures is in the lateral relation of the optic chiasma?
    a) lamina terminalis
    b) internal carotid artery
    c) tuber cinerium
    d) posterior perforated substance
1500. Complete the sentence—Fibres from the nasal half of each retina
    a) pass into the ipsilateral optic tract only.
    b) cross to the contralateral optic tract only.
    c) pass into both optic tracts.
    d) pass to the opposite retina.
1501. The third ventricle is the derivative of which of the primitive brain vesicle?
    a) forebrain
    b) midbrain
    c) hindbrain
    d) forebrain & midbrain
1502. All of the following parts of diencephalon form the wall of third ventricle **except**
    a) hypothalamus
    b) thalamus
    c) metathalamus
    d) epithalamus
1503. Which boundary of third ventricle contains the tela choroidea?
    a) lateral wall
    b) floor
    c) rostral boundary
    d) roof

1504. Artery supplying the choroid plexus of the third ventricle is a branch of
   a) anterior cerebral
   b) middle cerebral
   c) posterior cerebral
   d) internal corotid
1505. Posterior boundary of interpeduncular fossa of brain is formed by
   a) optic chiasma
   b) optic tracts
   c) cerebral peduncles
   d) pons
1506. All of the following structures lie in the interpeduncular fossa of brain **except**
   a) mammillary bodies
   b) tuber cinerium
   c) epiphysis cerebri
   d) posterior perforated substance
1507. Each cerebral hemisphere has all of the following structures **except**
   a) cortex
   b) white matter
   c) basal nuclei
   d) thalamus
1508. Surfaces of cerebral hemispheres are smooth upto
   a) the end of third foetal month
   b) the end of ninth foetal month
   c) third month after birth
   d) ninth month after birth
1509. Cerebral sulci developing along the zones separating areas differing in structure and function are termed as
   a) axial
   b) limiting
   c) operculated
   d) secondary
1510. Which of the following sulci of the cerebral cortex is a limiting sulcus?
   a) central
   b) lateral
   c) calcarine
   d) parieto-occipital
1511. 'Calcarine sulcus'·is the example of which of the following sulci?
   a) limiting
   b) axial
   c) operculated
   d) secondary
1512. Which of the following sulcus of cerebral cortex is 'operculated sulcus'?
   a) central
   b) calcarine
   c) parietooccipital
   d) lunate
1513. Which of the following sulcus is associated with the development of the corpus callosum?
   a) collateral
   b) calcarine
   c) parietoccipital
   d) central
1514. Which of the following sulcus of cerebral cortex is the example of secondary sulcus?
   a) lateral
   b) central
   c) calcarine
   d) lunate

Chapter IX
Head, Face, Neck and Nervous System

1515. Which of the following sulci of the cerebral cortex is the example of complete sulcus?
 a) central
 b) calcarine
 c) lateral
 d) parietooccipital

1516. How much area of the human cerebral cortex is obscured by sulci and gyri?
 a) one fourth
 b) half
 c) two thirds
 d) one third

1517. Which of the following statements regarding the human brain is/are misleading?
 a) a large increase in cortical area entails a lesser change in cranial capacity
 b) high intelligence is associated with great complexity of its convolutional pattern
 c) brain size is associated with cerebral abilities
 d) all of the above

1518. Which of the following arteries lies in the floor of lateral sulcus of cerebrum?
 a) interior cerebral
 b) middle cerebral
 c) posterior cerebral
 d) internal carotid

1519. Venous sinus contained in the cerebral lateral sulcus is
 a) sphenoparietal
 b) superior petrosal
 c) cavernous
 d) sigmoid

1520. Length of lateral sulcus of cerebrum is
 a) 5 cm
 b) 7 cm
 c) 9 cm
 d) 11 cm

1521. The starting point of the central sulcus on the superomedial border of cerebrum coincides with a point midway between
 a) nasion and inion
 b) bregma and lambda
 c) nasion and lambda
 d) bregma and inion

1522. The general direction of the central sulcus of cerebrum makes an angle with the median plane of about
 a) 20°
 b) 70°
 c) 90°
 d) 170°

1523. Sulcus that demarcates the primary motor and somtosensory areas of the cortex is
 a) lateral
 b) parietooccipital
 c) central
 d) calcarine

1524. Cortex giving origin to most of the corticospinal fibres is
 a) precentral
 b) postcentral
 c) cingulate
 d) prefrontal

1525. Cortical gyrus on which the 'speech area of Broca' lies is
   a) superior frontal
   b) middle frontal
   c) inferior frontal
   d) precentral

1526. Inferior end of precentral gyrus is continuous with
   a) par opercularis
   b) pars triangularis
   c) pars orbitalis
   d) temporal operculum

1527. An arbitary line limiting the temporal lobe posteriorly extends from the preoccipital notch to
   a) posterior end of lateral sulcus
   b) a point of meeting of parietooccipital sulcus and superomedial margin
   c) lower end of central sulcus
   d) lower end of post-central sulcus

1528. Which surface of the temporal lobe of the brain bear the transverse temporal gyri?
   a) upper
   b) lower
   c) medial
   d) lateral

1529. Functionally the anterior temporal gyrus of the cerebrum is
   a) visual
   b) somatic sensory
   c) gustatory
   d) auditory

1530. The anterior part of the inferior parietal lobule of cerebrum is known as
   a) supramarginal gyrus
   b) angular gyrus
   c) arcus temporooccipitalis
   d) arcus parietooccipitalis

1531. Angular gyrus of the cerebrum is believed to be concerned with the
   a) sensory speech
   b) visual element in stereognosis
   c) taste
   d) smell

1532. Which of the following areas is buried deeply in the lunate sulcus?
   a) striate
   b) peristriate
   c) parastriate
   d) none of the above

1533. Gyrus ambiens belongs to which fo the following part of the cerebral cortex?
   a) parietal lobe
   b) medial surface
   c) temporal lobe
   d) insula

1534. Which of the following structures lies in the central part of floor of the longitudinal fissure of cerebrum?
   a) vermis
   b) interthalamic adhesion
   c) anterior commissure
   d) corpus callosum

1535. The rostrum of corpus callosum as it passess back continues with
   a) anterior commissure
   b) lamina terminalis
   c) fornix
   d) genu

1536. Rounded posterior extremity of corpus callosum is known as
   a) rostrum
   b) splenium
   c) genu
   d) trunk
1537. Which of the following is the prehippocampal rudiment?
   a) paraterminal gyrus
   b) parolfactory gyrus
   c) lamina terminalis
   d) gyrus rectus
1538. Anterior region of the medial surface of cerebral hemisphere is divided into outer and inner zones by
   a) horizontal fissure
   b) circular sulcus
   c) cingulate sulcus
   d) collateral sulcus
1539. Cortical area which exercises control over defecation and micturation is
   a) precentral gyrus
   b) cingulate gyrus
   c) medial frontal gyrus
   d) paracentral lobule
1540. Which of following gyri separates the parietooccipital and calcarine sulci deeply?
   a) parahippocampal
   b) cuneate
   c) lingual
   d) precuneate
1541. The thickness of human cerebral cortex varies from
   a) 0.15 to 0.45 mm
   b) 1.5 to 4.5 mm
   c) 1.5 mm to 4.5 cm
   d) 1.5 to 4.5 cm
1542. Which of the following cells of the cerebral cortex are considered to be modified pyramidal neurons?
   a) basket
   b) neurogliaform
   c) cells of Martinotti
   d) pleomorphic
1543. The projection axons from the cerebral cortex to the subcortical centres originate mainly from
   a) pyramidal cells
   b) stellate nerve cells
   c) horizontal cells
   d) cells of Martinotti
1544. Nerve axon fibres crossing the midline from one cerebral hemisphere to another are know as
   a) association
   b) commisural
   c) projection
   d) arcuate
1545. Which of the following cells of the cerebral cortex are often called as granule cells?
   a) pyramidal
   b) horizontal
   c) pleomorphic
   d) stellate
1546. Which of the following cells appear in greatest abdudance in lamina II and IV of cerebral cortex?
   a) stellate
   b) pyramidal
   c) horizontal
   d) pleomorphic

1547. Which of the following laminae of the cerebral cortex contains the external band of Baillarger?
   a) external granular
   b) pyramidal
   c) internal granular
   d) ganglionic

1548. Which of the following neuronal type is prominent in the agranular type of cerebral cortex?
   a) stellate
   b) pyramidal
   c) horizontal
   d) cells of Martinotti

1549. Which of the following representative variant of the cortical structure is visuopsychic area?
   a) frontal
   b) parietal
   c) temporal
   d) polar

1550. Structurally, which of the cortical type is often equated with motor area?
   a) granular
   b) agranular
   c) both a & b
   d) none

1551. A typical granular cortex appears in all of the following cortical areas **except**
   a) postcentral gyrus
   b) striate area
   c) superior temporal gyrus
   d) precentral gyrus

1552. The external band of Baillarger of the cerebral cortex is well defined as the stria of Gennari in
   a) frontal area
   b) temporal area
   c) striate cortex
   d) parietal cortex

1553. Which of the following type is the thinnest part of cerebral cortex?
   a) polar
   b) frontal
   c) parietal
   d) temporal

1554. Which of the following cortical area is known as supplementary motor area?
   a) precentral gyrus
   b) postcentral gyrus
   c) medial cerebral surface
   d) prefrontal cortex

1555. Cortical area featuring almost complete absence of granular layer is
   a) precentral
   b) postcentral
   c) visual
   d) auditory

1556. The giant pyramidal cells of Betz vary in height from
   a) 0.3 to 0.12 micron
   b) 3 to 12 micron
   c) 30 to 120 micron
   d) 300 to 1200 micron

1557. Conjugate ocular movements are elicited by stimulation of Brodmann area
   a) 4
   b) 8
   c) 44
   d) 18

58. The second speech area of Wernicke extends more extensively in which of the following lobes?
    a) frontal
    b) parietal
    c) temporal
    d) occipital
59. 'Astereognosis' is associated with damage to which of the following lobe?
    a) frontal
    b) pariental
    c) temporal
    d) occipital
60. Which of the following gyri of the cerebral cortex contains the vestibular area?
    a) precentral
    b) postcentral
    c) superior temporal
    d) angular
61. The septum pellucidum is attached above to the
    a) fornix
    b) lower surface of trunk of corpus callosum
    c) upper surface of trunk of corpus callosum
    d) upper surface of thalamus
62. Bulb of posterior horn of lateral ventricle is formed by
    a) forceps major
    b) forceps minor
    c) tapetum
    d) calcarine sulcus
63. The two lateral ventricles are almost completely separated by
    a) falx cerebri
    b) corpus callosum
    c) septum pellucidum
    d) thalamus
64. All of the following structures form the floor of central part of lateral ventricle **except**
    a) caudate nucleus
    b) superior surface of thalamus
    c) stria medullaris thalami
    d) thalamostriate vein
65. A narrow groove along the medial border of the caudate nucleus in the floor of central part of lateral ventricle contains
    a) stria medullaris thalami
    b) lamina terminalis
    c) longitudinal stria
    d) stria terminalis
66. The fissure between the fornicial edge and reciprocal groove on the superior surface of thalamus is
    a) transverse
    b) longitudinal
    c) lateral
    d) choroid
67. Roof of central part of lateral ventricle is formed by
    a) corona radiata
    b) corpus callosum
    c) septum pellucidum
    d) tela choroidea
68. Roof and lateral wall of posterior horn of lateral ventricle is formed by
    a) corpus callosum
    b) tapetum
    c) bulbs of posterior horn
    d) calcar avis

1569. Roof of the inferior horn of lateral ventricle is formed by all of following **except**
   a) hippocampus
   b) tapetum
   c) tail of caudate nucleus
   d) stria terminalis

1570. Inferior part of the choroid fissure lies between
   a) fornix and inferior surface of thalamus
   b) stria terminalis and fimbria
   c) fornix and superior surface of thalamus
   d) caudate nucleus and collateral eminence

1571. Fibres connecting the cerebral cortex to the subcortical gray matter in both directions are
   a) projection
   b) commissural
   c) long association
   d) short association

1572. Fasciculus following a sharply curved course across the stem of lateral sulcus is known as
   a) frontooccipital
   b) inferior longitudinal
   c) cingulum
   d) uncinate

1573. Neuronal fibres forming corona radiata are
   a) projection fibres
   b) commissural fibres
   c) association fibres
   d) nonspecific fibres

1574. Medial aspect of corona radiata is separated from the lateral ventricle by
   a) frontooccipital fasciculus
   b) superior longitudinal fasciculus
   c) unciate fasciculus
   d) fibres of corpus callosum

1575. The genu of the internal capsule is usually regarded as containing which of the following fibres?
   a) corticopontine
   b) corticonuclear
   c) corticospinal
   d) corticorubral

1576. Which part of internal capsule contains frontopontine fibres?
   a) anterior limb
   b) genu
   c) retrolentiform part
   d) posterior limb

1577. All of the following fibres are contained in the retrolentiform part of the internal capsule **except**
   a) occipitopontine
   b) occipitocollicular
   c) frontopontine
   d) optic radiation

1578. Optic radiation fibres arise in
   a) medial geniculale body
   b) lateral geniculate body
   c) superior colliculus
   d) inferior colliculus

1579. The sublentiform part of the internal capsule contains all of the following fibres **except**
   a) temporopontine
   b) parietopontine
   c) occipitopontine
   d) acoustic radiation

Chapter IX — Head, Face, Neck and Nervous System 157

80. Acoustic radiation fibres originate from
    a) medial geniculate body
    b) lateral geniculate body
    c) superior colliculus
    d) inferior colliculus

81. All of the following structures are included in basal nuclei **except**
    a) amygdaloid complex
    b) subthalamus
    c) caudate nucleus
    d) lentiform nucleus

82. All of the following structures are the part of corpus striatum **except**
    a) putamen
    b) claustrum
    c) globus pallidus
    d) caudate nucleus

83. Body of caudate nucleus is separated from the globus pallidus by
    a) claustrum
    b) occipitofrontal fasciculus
    c) superior longitudinal fasciculus
    d) internal capsule

84. Between the claustrum and the insular cortex is present the
    a) putamen
    b) internal capsule
    c) external capsule
    d) extreme capsule

85. Which of the following fibres are involved in the Parkinsonian tremor?
    a) corticostriate
    b) nigrostriate
    c) thalamostriate
    d) striatonigral

86. The pallidofugal system contains all of the following paths **except**
    a) dorsal longitudinal fasciculus
    b) fasciaculus thalamicus
    c) ansa lenticularis
    d) fasciculus subthalamicus

87. An average human male adult's brain weighs about
    a) 500 gm
    b) 1000 gm
    c) 1500 gm
    d) 2000 gm

88. In an average adult human, brain : body weight ratio is
    a) 1 : 12
    b) 1 : 25
    c) 1 : 50
    d) 1 : 80

89. Arterial supply to the medial and inferior surface of the cerebral hemisphere is from
    a) anterior cerebral
    b) middle cerebral
    c) posterior cerebral
    d) all of the above

90. Charcot's artery of cerebral haemorrhage is a branch of
    a) anterior cerebral
    b) posterior cerebral
    c) middle meningeal
    d) middle cerebral

91. All of the following arteries supply the midbrain **except**
    a) superior cerebellar
    b) middle cerebral
    c) posterior cerebral
    d) basillar

92. Pons is supplied by all of the following arteries **except**
    a) superior cerebellar
    b) basillar
    c) anterior inferior cerebellar
    d) posterior inferior cerebellar

1593. Artery supplying the choroid plexus of the fourth ventricle is
   a) anterior inferior cerebellar
   b) posterior cerebral
   c) posterior inferior cerebellar
   d) middle cerebral

1594. Arterial supply to median zone of optic chiasma is from
   a) anterior cerebral
   b) middle cerebral
   c) internal carotid
   d) middle meningeal

1595. Vein formed by union of thalamostriate and chorodial veins is
   a) anterior cerebral
   b) deep middle cerebral
   c) internal cerebral
   d) basal

1596. Lymphatics are absent in which of the following body organ?
   a) kidney
   b) brain
   c) lung
   d) liver

1597. The falx cerebri splits to enclose all of the following blood sinuses except
   a) straight
   b) occipital
   c) superior sagittal
   d) inferior sagittal

1598. Which of the following folds of dura mater is involved in the formation of 'trigeminal cave'?
   a) falx cerebri
   b) falx cerebelli
   c) tentorium cerebelli
   d) diaphragma sellae

1599. Which of the following dural fold forms the roof of the hypophyseal fossa?
   a) tentorium cerebelli
   b) falx cerebri
   c) diaphragma sellae
   d) falx cerebelli

1600. A small central opening in the diaphragma sellae transmits the
   a) internal carotid artery
   b) infundibulum of pituitary gland
   c) optic chiasma
   d) basillar vein

1601. All of the following structures pierce the roof of the cavernous sinus except
   a) internal carotid artery
   b) abducent nerve
   c) oculomotor nerve
   d) trochlear nerve

1602. It is impossible to differentiate the meninges from one another within the
   a) longitudinal fissure of brain
   b) foramen magnum
   c) sella turcica
   d) anterior cranial fossa

1603. Which of the following cranial nerves is the most authentic source of cerebral dural innervation?
   a) trigeminal
   b) vestibulochochlear
   c) glossopharyngeal
   d) accessory

1604. Nervus spinosus is a branch of
   a) maxillary nerve
   b) mandibular nerve
   c) ophthalmic nerve
   d) first cervical nerve

Chapter IX Head, Face, Neck and Nervous System

1605. Which of the following spaces contain cerebrospinal fluid?
   a) subdural
   b) epidural
   c) subarachnoid
   d) all of the above

1606. The cerebral part of arachnoid matter does not enter the sulci or fissure **with the exception** of
   a) central sulcus
   b) lateral sulcus
   c) transverse fissure
   d) longitudinal fissure

1607. Which of the following subarachnoid cistern contains the great cerebral vein?
   a) cisterna ambiens
   b) pontine cistern
   c) cerebellomedullary cistern
   d) interpeduncular cistern

1608. The number of openings connecting the subarachnoid space with the ventricles is
   a) one
   b) two
   c) three
   d) four

1609. The spinal subarachnoid space ends below at the lower border of which vertebra?
   a) twelfth thoracic
   b) first lumbar
   c) second sacral
   d) fifth sacral

1610. In the cerebrospinal fluid brain weighs only
   a) 50 gm
   b) 150 gm
   c) 500 gm
   d) 1500 gm

1611. Specimens of cerebrospinal fluid are obtained through the interval between vertebral spines
   a) twelfth thoracic and first lumbar
   b) first and second lumbar
   c) third and fourth lumbar
   d) second and third sacral

1612. In human body number of pairs of spinal nerves are
   a) 30
   b) 31
   c) 32
   d) 33

1613. Connective tissue sheath covering the fasciculus of the nerve fibres is
   a) epineurium
   b) endoneurium
   c) perineurium
   d) endomycium

1614. 'Nervi nervorum' are
   a) blood vessels supplying a nerve
   b) nerves supplying the blood vessels of the larger nerve
   c) nerve supplying a bigger nerve
   d) none of the above

1615. Aggregation of the nerve cell bodies in the central nervous system is known as a
   a) tract
   b) ganglia
   c) nucleus
   d) nerve

1616. All of the following cranial nerves are associated with a ganglia **except**
   a) trigeminal
   b) abducent
   c) facial
   d) glossopharyngeal

1617. Which of the following ganglia **does not show** the presence of synaptic glomeruli?
   a) prevertebral
   b) paravertebral
   c) parasympathetic
   d) spinal

1618. Which of the following ganglia show presence of the synapse?
   a) geniculate
   b) otic
   c) trigeminal
   d) spinal

1619. Olfactory nerves serving the sense of smell have their cells of origin in the
   a) olfactory bulb
   b) olfactory trigone
   c) olfactory mucosa of nose
   d) pyriform cortex

1620. Which of the following nerves are unique in having the peripheral origin of their neurons in the ectoderm?
   a) olfactory
   b) optic
   c) oculomotor
   d) trigeminal

1621. Subarachnoid space is communicated with the tissue space in the mucosa of
   a) mouth cavity
   b) nasal cavity
   c) middle ear
   d) pharynx

1622. All of the following statements regarding the nervi terminales are true **except**
   a) it is considered to be the thirteenth cranial nerve
   b) its fibre are mainly myelinated
   c) it lies medial to the olfactory tract
   d) it passess to the nasal mucosa

1623. Most of the nerve fibres of the optic nerve originate from
   a) rods and cones of retina
   b) retinal ganglionic neurons
   c) superior colliculus
   d) lateral geniculate body

1624. Developmentally, which of the following nerves is the outgrowth of the brain?
   a) olfactory
   b) optic
   c) vestibulocochlear
   d) facial

1625. Nerve fibres of which of the following nerves are covered by oligodendrocytes?
   a) optic
   b) olfactory
   c) trigeminal
   d) vestibulocochlear

1626. The ciliary ganglia lies between the optic nerve and the
   a) lateral rectus
   b) medial rectus
   c) superior oblique
   d) inferior rectus

Chapter IX Head, Face, Neck and Nervous System **161**

627. In the optic canal the relation of the optic nerve to the ophthalmic artery is
   a) superomedial
   b) inferomedial
   c) superolateral
   d) inferolateral

628. Which of the following nerve crosses the optic nerve from above in the orbital cavity?
   a) frontal
   b) superior division of the oculomotor
   c) abducent
   d) nasociliary

629. All of the following structures lie above the optic nerve in its intracranial part **except**
   a) internal carotid artery
   b) olfactory tract
   c) gyrus rectus
   d) anterior cerebral artery

630. The pial plexus supplying arterial blood to the optic nerve is formed by all of the following arteries **except**
   a) infraorbital
   b) ophthalmic
   c) central retinal
   d) superior hypophyseal

631. Increase in CSF in the general subarachnoid space easily leads to neuritis in which of the following nerves?
   a) olfactory
   b) optic
   c) trigeminal
   d) vestibulocochlear

632. All of the following extraocular muscles are supplied by the oculomotor nerve **except**
   a) superior oblique
   b) inferior oblique
   c) medial rectus
   d) inferior rectus

633. Which of the following nerve is associated with the ciliary ganglia?
   a) optic
   b) oculomotor
   c) trochlear
   d) abducent

634. Fibres of which of the following nerve pierce the red nucleus?
   a) optic
   b) oculomotor
   c) trochlear
   d) trigeminal

635. Somata of the afferent fibres contained in the oculomotor nerve lie in the
   a) oculomotor nucleus
   b) Edinger-Westphal nucleus
   c) ciliary ganglia
   d) trigeminal ganglia

636. Preganglionic parasympathetic fibres of the oculomotor nerve originate from neurons of
   a) ciliary ganglia
   b) accessory oculomotor nucleus
   c) trigeminal ganglia
   d) main oculomotor nucleus

1637. Connections of the oculomotor nuclei include all of the following **except**
   a) corticonuclear tract
   b) medial longitudinal fasciculus
   c) tectobular tract
   d) lateral lemniscus

1638. Which of the following nerves passes through the tendinous ring of the superior orbital fissure?
   a) frontal
   b) oculomotor
   c) lacrimal
   d) trochlear

1639. All of the following nerves pass through the tendinous ring of the superior orbital fissure **except**
   a) nasociliary
   b) occulomotor
   c) trochlear
   d) abducent

1640. The inferior ramus of the oculomotor nerve supplies all of the following extraocular muscles **except**
   a) superior rectus
   b) medial rectus
   c) inferior rectus
   d) inferior oblique

1641. The branches of the inferior ramus of the oculomotor nerve enter the muscles on their ocular surface, **except that to**
   a) inferior oblique
   b) inferior rectus
   c) medial rectus
   d) none of the above

1642. Nerve to which of the following extraocular muscles give rise to a branch to the ciliary ganglion?
   a) rectus medialis
   b) rectus lateralis
   c) superior rectus
   d) inferior oblique

1643. Somata of which of the following neurons are present in the ciliary ganglion?
   a) sympathetic
   b) parasympathetic
   c) sensory
   d) all of the above

1644. Which of the following nerve gives rise to the sensory root of the ciliary ganglia?
   a) nasociliary
   b) frontal
   c) lacrimal
   d) infraorbital

1645. Somata of the postganglionic sympathetic fibres of short ciliary nerves lie in the
   a) ciliary ganglion
   b) trigeminal ganglion
   c) superior cervical ganglion
   d) pterygopalatine ganglion

1646. Complete severance of the oculomotor nerve leads to all of the following sequelae **except**
   a) ptosis
   b) proptosis
   c) pupillary constriction
   d) lateral strabismus

1647. Which of the following muscles is supplied by the trochlear nerve?
   a) superior rectus
   b) inferior oblique
   c) superior oblique
   d) lateral rectus

Chapter IX — Head, Face, Neck and Nervous System

1648. Trochlear nerve nucleus receives connections from all of the following **except** the
    a) corticonuclear tracts
    b) medial longitudinal fasciculus
    c) tectobulbar tract
    d) pretectal nuclei

1649. Which of the following is the only nerve emerging dorsally from the brain stem?
    a) oculomotor
    b) abducent
    c) trochlear
    d) trigeminal

1650. Fibres of which of the following nerve decussate before emerging out from the brain stem?
    a) oculomotor
    b) trochlear
    c) abducent
    d) facial

1651. Interruption of the trochlear nerve produces diplopia mainly while looking
    a) upwards
    b) downwards
    c) medially
    d) laterally

1652. Which of the following divisions of the trigeminal nerve carries motor fibres?
    a) ophthalmic
    b) maxillary
    c) mandibular
    d) none of the above

1653. Neurons of which of the following nucleus of trigeminal nerve are the only sensory neurons with somata in the central nervous system?
    a) principal sensory
    b) mesencephalic
    c) spinal
    d) all of the above

1654. Which of the following nuclei occupies the position of the branchial efferent column in the brain stem?
    a) oculomotor
    b) trochlear
    c) abducent
    d) motor trigeminal

1655. All of the following are the branches of the ophthalmic nerve **except**
    a) frontal
    b) infraorbital
    c) nasociliary
    d) lacrimal

1656. Which of the following branches of the ophthalmic nerve adhere to the trochlear nerve?
    a) frontal
    b) nasociliary
    c) recurrent meningeal
    d) lacrimal

1657. The lacrimal nerve receives lacrimal secretomotor fibres from
    a) ciliary ganglion
    b) zygomaticotemporal nerve
    c) zygomaticofacial nerve
    d) nasociliary nerve

1658. All of the following are the branches of the nasociliary nerve **except**
    a) anterior ethmoidal
    b) posterior ethmoidal
    c) zygomaticofacial
    d) infratrochlear

1659. Which of the following nerves is functionally connected with the pterygopalatine ganglion?
   a) oculomotor
   b) maxillary
   c) glossopharyngeal
   d) facial

1660. Which of the following ganglia is closely related to the maxillary nerve?
   a) otic
   b) pterygopalatine
   c) ciliary
   d) submandibular

1661. The parasympathetic root of the pterygopalatine ganglia is
   a) oculomotor nerve-inferior division
   b) nerve to pterygoid canal
   c) nasociliary nerve
   d) chorda tympani

1662. Which of the following branches of the maxillary nerve carries the parasympathetic fibres?
   a) palpebral
   b) zygomatic
   c) posterior superior alveolar
   d) middle superior alveolar

1663. Fibres contained in the deep petrosal nerve are
   a) sympathetic
   b) parasympathetic
   c) sensory
   d) all of the above

1664. Somata of the fibres contained in deep petrosal nerve lie in
   a) pterygopalatine ganglion
   b) trigeminal ganglion
   c) superior cervical ganglion
   d) thoracic spinal cord

1665. Somata of the fibres conveying taste impulses from the palate are located in
   a) nucleus solitarius
   b) glossopharyngeal ganglion
   c) facial ganglion
   d) vagal ganglia

1666. Muscle supplied by the branch of mandibular nerve given before its division into anterior and posterior divisions is
   a) medial pterygoid
   b) lateral pterygoid
   c) temporalis
   d) masseter

1667. Which of the following branches of the anterior division of mandibular nerve is sensory?
   a) buccal
   b) masseteric
   c) deep temoporal
   d) all of the above

1668. Nerve passing through the mandibular notch is
   a) auriculotemporal
   b) masseteric
   c) buccal
   d) inferior alveolar

1669. Which of the following nerves usually has two roots of origin?
   a) masseteric
   b) auriculotemporal
   c) inferior alveolar
   d) buccal

Chapter IX   Head, Face, Neck and Nervous System   165

1670. All of the following are the branches of the posterior trunk of the mandibular nerve **except**
   a) lingual
   b) buccal
   c) inferior alveolar
   d) auriculotemporal

1671. Nerve carrying postganglionic parasymapathetic fibres of the parotid gland is
   a) facial
   b) lingual
   c) auriculotemporal
   d) inferior alveolar

1672. Which of the following cranial nerves carries the preganglionic parasympathetic fibres of the parotid gland?
   a) facial
   b) oculomotor
   c) vagal
   d) glossopharyngeal

1673. Somata of postganglionic secretomotor fibres to parotid gland lie in
   a) pterygopalatine ganglion
   b) otic ganglion
   c) geniculate ganglion
   d) glossopharyngeal ganglion

1674. Preganglionic parasympathetic neurons to parotid gland originate from
   a) thoracic spinal cord
   b) superior salivatory nucleus
   c) inferior salivatory nucleus
   d) nucleus ambiguus

1675. Which of the following nerves carries the preganglionic parasympathetic fibres from inferior salivary nucleus?
   a) chorda tymapani
   b) greater petrosal nerve
   c) deep petrosal nerve
   d) lesser petrosal nerve

1676. Lingual nerve is the branch of
   a) glossopharyngeal nerve
   b) facial nerve
   c) mandibular nerve
   d) hypoglossal nerve

1677. Which of the following nerves gives rise to the chorda tympani nerve?
   a) glossopharyngeal
   b) vagus
   c) facial
   d) lingual

1678. Nerve carrying preganglion parasympathetic fibres to the submandibular ganglion is
   a) lesser petrosal
   b) greater petrosal
   c) chorda tympani
   d) deep petrosal

1679. Lingual nerve can be pressed against a bone inside the mouth near the roots of the*
   a) third upper molar
   b) second upper molar
   c) third lower molar
   d) second lower molar

1680. Lingual nerve carries postganglionic parasympathetic fibres from ? ganglion?
   a) otic
   b) pterygopalatine
   c) submandibular
   d) ciliary

1681. Which of the following nerves passes between the sphenomandibular ligament and the mandibular ramus?
   a) lingual
   b) chorda tympani
   c) inferior alveolar
   d) buccal

1682. All of the following nerves pass between medial pterygoid and the mandibular ramus **except**
   a) inferior alveolar
   b) mylohyoid
   c) lingual
   d) buccal

1683. Which of the following nerves passes through the mandibular foramen?
   a) buccal
   b) inferior alveolar
   c) auriculotemporal
   d) chorda tympani

1684. Nerve piercing the sphenomandibular ligament is
   a) inferior alveolar
   b) lingual
   c) mylohyoid
   d) buccal

1685. Loss of taste in the anterior two thirds of tongue occurs because of lesion of
   a) facial nerve near the geniculate ganglion
   b) chorda tympani nerve
   c) lingual nerve below its junction with chorda tympani nerve
   d) any of the above

1686. 'Ophthalmic neuralgia' is often associated with all of the following **except**
   a) acute glaucoma
   b) frontal sinusitis
   c) maxillary sinusitis
   d) ethmoidal sinusitis

1687. Disease of which of the following regions causes referred pain in ear?
   a) maxillary sinus
   b) cornea
   c) mandibular teeth
   d) frontal sinus

1688. In order to ease pain due to a lingual carcinoma, a nerve occasionally divided is
   a) inferior alveolar
   b) buccal
   c) lingual
   d) chorda tympani

1689. To ease the pain of ophthalmic neuralgia, the preferred operation is
   a) injection of trigeminal ganglion with alcohol
   b) division of sensory root behind the ganglion
   c) division of ophthalmic nerve intracranially
   d) division of spinal tract of trigeminal, where it is most superficial

1690. Section of the spinal tract of trigeminal 4.5 mm caudal to the obex preserves most of the nerve fibres of
   a) ophthalmic nerve
   b) maxillary nerve
   c) mandibular nerve
   d) none of the above

1691. Which of the following nerves supplies lateral rectus muscle?
   a) trochlear
   b) oculomotor
   c) ophthalmic
   d) abducent

692. Which of the following nerves emerge through the sulcus between pons and pyramids of medulla oblongata?
    a) facial
    b) vestibulocochlear
    c) abducent
    d) glossopharyngeal
693. Which of the following nerves is most liable to damage in conditions producing raised intracranial pressure?
    a) abducent   b) facial   c) oculomotor   d) trigeminal
694. Damage to which of the following nerves lead to the convergent squint?
    a) oculomotor
    b) trochlear
    c) abducent
    d) all of the above
695. The glossopharyngeal nerve carries preganglionic parasympathetic innervation to which of the following gland?
    a) parotid
    b) submandibular
    c) sublingual
    d) lacrimal
696. Nerve carrying gustatory fibres from the soft palate is
    a) glossopharyngeal
    b) vagus
    c) facial
    d) accessory
697. Which of the following nerves carries the gustatory fibres from the presulcal area of tongue?
    a) greater petrosal
    b) chorda tympani
    c) glossopharyngeal
    d) vagus
698. Course of which of the following nerves exhibits neurobiotaxis?
    a) abducent
    b) oculomotor
    c) trochlear
    d) facial
699. Nucleus of which of the following nerves is reputedly supplied by the aberrant pyramidal fibres descending in the medial lemniscus?
    a) trochlear
    b) hypoglossal
    c) abducent
    d) facial
700. Contralateral corticonuclear fibres end in the part of the facial nerve nucleus innervating the muscles of
    a) whole face
    b) lower part of face
    c) periorbital region
    d) periorbital region and forehead
701. Corticonuclear projection to neurons for muscles around eyes and forehead is
    a) bilateral
    b) ipsilateral only
    c) contralateral only
    d) doubtful
702. All of the following nerves are attached between the olive and the inferior cerebellar peduncle at the cerebellopontine angle **except**
    a) vestibulocochlear
    b) abducent
    c) facial
    d) nervus intermedius

1703. The nervus intermedius contains the centripetal processes of the unipolar neurons in the
   a) trigeminal ganglion
   b) geniculate ganglion
   c) glossopharyngeal ganglion
   d) vagal ganglion

1704. The nervus intermedius contains all of the following fibres **except**
   a) centripetal processes of unipolar neurons in the geniculate ganglion
   b) somatic afferent fibres from auricular concha
   c) efferent preganglionic parasympathetic fibres
   d) branchial efferent

1705. Which of the following nerves has transparotid course?
   a) glossopharyngeal
   b) accessory
   c) facial
   d) hypoglossal

1706. Nerve lying about 2 cm deep to the middle of anterior border of mastoid process is
   a) mandibular
   b) auriculotemporal
   c) chorda tympani
   d) facial

1707. The greater petrosal nerve contains mainly the taste fibres from.
   a) palatal mucosa
   b) epiglottis
   c) posterior third of tongue
   d) anterior two third of tongue

1708. Which of the following ganglia receives the preganglionic parasympathetic fibres from the greater petrosal nerve?
   a) otic
   b) pterygopalatine
   c) submandibular
   d) ciliary

1709. Nerves joining to form the nerve of the pterygoid conal are
   a) lesser and greater petrosal
   b) lesser and deep petrosal
   c) deep petrosal and chorda tympani
   d) greater and deep petrosal

1710. Deep petrosal nerve originates from
   a) mandibular nerve
   b) facial nerve
   c) glossopharyngeal nerve
   d) internal carotid sympathetic plexus

1711. Somata of which of the following neurons are located in the pterygopalatine ganglion?
   a) somatic afferent
   b) gustatory
   c) postganglionic parasympathetic
   d) postganglionic sympathetic

1712. Which of the following fibres pass without interruption through the pterygopalatine ganglion?
   a) gustatory
   b) somatic afferent
   c) sympathetic
   d) all of the above

713. All of the following branches are given by the facial nerve at its exit from the stylomastoid foramen **except**
    a) digastric
    b) stylohyoid
    c) chorda tympani
    d) posterior auricular
714. Submandibular ganglion is functionally connected with which of the following nerves?
    a) glossopharyngeal
    b) facial
    c) vagus
    d) oculomotor
715. All of the following are the peripheral parasympathetic ganglia **except**
    a) geniculate
    b) otic
    c) pterygopalatine
    d) ciliary
716. The sympathetic root to the submandibular ganglion is derived from the plexus on the
    a) external carotid artery
    b) facial artery
    c) internal carotid artery
    d) lingual artery
717. Movements of which part of face are usually severely affected in the supranuclear facial paralysis?
    a) upper half
    b) lower half
    c) upper and lower both the halves
    d) none of the above
718. All of the following statements regarding the supranuclear facial paralysis are correct **except**
    a) it is usually associated with hemiplegia
    b) movements in upper part of face are more severely affected
    c) emotional expression is little affected
    d) electrical reactions of affected muscles are unaltered
719. Facial muscle paralysis due to complete lesion of the facial nucleus is
    a) ipsilateral upper and lower half
    b) ipsilateral lower half only
    c) contralateral
    d) bilateral
720. Which of the following vestibular nucleus forms the vestibulospinal tract?
    a) superior
    b) lateral
    c) inferior
    d) medial
721. Which of the following ganglia contains the somata of the cochlear nerve fibres?
    a) spiral
    b) vestibular
    c) geniculate
    d) trigeminal
722. 'Trapezoid body' of pons is formed by decussation of contralateral
    a) pontocerebellar fibres
    b) second neuron fibres in the auditory pathway
    c) second neuron fibres in the proprioceptive pathway
    d) second neuron fibres in vestibular pathway

1723. Which of the lemniscus is formed by the ascending second order neurons of the auditory pathway?
   a) lateral
   b) medial
   c) spinal
   d) trigeminal

1724. Commissural fibres link the two auditory pathways at the level of
   a) cochlear nuclei
   b) trapezoid nuclei
   c) inferior colliculus
   d) medial geniculate body

1725. Muscle supplied by the glossopharyngeal nerve is
   a) stylopharyngeus
   b) palatopharyngeus
   c) palatoglossus
   d) styloglossus

1726. Gland receiving the parasympathetic secretomotor fibres from the glossopharyngeal nerve is
   a) submandibular
   b) lacrimal
   c) parotid
   d) sublingual

1727. Glossopharyngeal nerve is gustatory to the
   a) palate
   b) epiglottis
   c) anterior two thirds of tongue
   d) posterior third of tongue

1728. Fibres concerned with taste sensation end in the nucleus
   a) solitarius
   b) ambiguus
   c) spinal trigeminal
   d) inferior salivatory

1729. Parasympathetic fibres of the glossopharyngeal nerve originate in
   a) nucleus ambiguus
   b) solitary nucleus
   c) inferior salivatory nucleus
   d) superior salivatory nucleus

1730. Nucleus giving rise to motor fibres of the glossopharyngeal nerve is
   a) solitary nucleus
   b) nucleus ambiguus
   c) dorsal vagal nucleus
   d) inferior salivatory nucleus

1731. Preganglionic parasympathetic fibres of the glossopharyngeal nerve terminate in which of the following ganglia?
   a) otic
   b) pterygopalatine
   c) ciliary
   d) submandibular

1732. Which of the following branches of the glossopharyngeal nerve carries the preganglionic parasympathetic fibres for the parotid gland?
   a) carotid
   b) tympanic
   c) pharyngeal
   d) tonsillar

1733. Which of the following nerves receives the postganglionic parasympathetic fibres from the otic ganglion?
   a) lesser petrosal
   b) auriculotemporal
   c) palatine
   d) pharyngeal

1734. Which of the following nerves passes between the superior and middle pharyngeal constrictors?
   a) glossopharyngeal
   b) hypoglossal
   c) superior laryngeal
   d) inferior laryngeal

Chapter IX Head, Face, Neck and Nervous System 171

735. Tympanic nerve plexus supplies branches to all of the following nerves **except**
    a) lesser petrosal
    b) greater petrosal
    c) chorda tympani
    d) nerves to mucosa of middle ear
736. Lesser petrosal nerve is the branch of
    a) glossopharyngeal nerve
    b) tympanic nerve plexus
    c) vagus nerve
    d) facial nerve
737. Pharyngeal nerve plexus receives contribution from all of the following nerves **except**
    a) facial
    b) vagus
    c) glossopharyngeal
    d) sympathetic trunk
738. Ganglion topographically related to the mandibular nerve, but functionally connected with the glossopharyngeal is
    a) otic
    b) pterygopalatine
    c) ciliary
    d) submandibular
739. Postrematic nerve of third branchial arch is
    a) facial
    b) glossopharyngeal
    c) superior laryngeal
    d) mandibular
740. Cranial nerve most extensive in its course and distribution is
    a) trigeminal
    b) accessory
    c) vagus
    d) glossopharyngeal
741. Which of the following nucleus gives rise to the general visceral efferent fibres of vagus?
    a) dorsal nucleus of vagus
    b) nucleus ambiguus
    c) nucleus solitarius
    d) inferior salivatory nucleus
742. Which of the following functional columns of brain stem is represented by the nucleus ambiguus?
    a) general visceral efferent
    b) general visceral afferent
    c) somatic afferent
    d) branchial efferent
743. Which of the following nerve pairs share a common arachnoid and dural sheath?
    a) vagus and accessory
    b) glossopharyngeal and vagus
    c) glossopharyngeal and accessory
    d) accessory and hypoglossal
744. The cranial accessory blends with the vagus
    a) before the superior ganglion of vagus
    b) between superior and inferior ganglia of vagus
    c) beyond the inferior ganglion of vagus
    d) at its emergence from the brain stem

1745. The preganglionic parasympathetic neurons of the vagus nerve terminate in which of the following ganglion?
 a) pterygopalatine
 b) inferior vagal
 c) superior vagal
 d) in the wall of target organ

1746. Both vagal ganglia contain the somata of all of the following fibres **except**
 a) somatic afferent
 b) special visceral afferent
 c) general visceral afferent
 d) parasympathetic postganglionic

1747. Superior vagal ganglion is
 a) cheifly somatic
 b) cheifly gustatory
 c) cheifly visceral
 d) all of the above

1748. Which of the following nerves descends vertically in the carotid sheath between internal jugular vein and internal carotid artery?
 a) glossopharyngeal
 b) vagus
 c) accessory
 d) hypoglossal

1749. Which of the following nerves is reponsible for an abnormal reflex known as 'ear cough'?
 a) trigeminal
 b) facial
 c) vagus
 d) glossopharyngeal

1750. Which part of the accessory nerve should be considered as part of the vagus nerve?
 a) cranial
 b) spinal
 c) cranial and spinal both
 d) none of the above

1751. The cranial part of accessory nerve originates from
 a) spinal nucleus
 b) nucleus ambiguus
 c) hypoglossal nucleus
 d) nucleus solitarius

1752. All of the following muscles are supplied by the fibres of cranial accessory nerve through vagus **except**
 a) tensor veli palatini
 b) musculus uvulae
 c) levator veli palatini
 d) palatoglossus

1753. **Except** tensor veli palatini, all of the muscles of soft palate are supplied by which of the following nerves?
 a) glossopharyngeal
 b) cranial part of accessory
 c) spinal part of accessory
 d) mandibular

1754. Which of the following muscles of soft palate is supplied by the mandibular nerve?
 a) levator veli palatini
 b) tensor veli palatini
 c) palatopharyngeus
 d) palatoglossus

1755. The 'spinal nucleus' of the accessory nerve descends in the anterior gray column of the spinal cord up to which spinal segment?
 a) first cervical
 b) fifth cervical
 c) seventh cervical
 d) first thoracic

Chapter IX Head, Face, Neck and Nervous System   173

1756. The spinal root of the accessory nerve enters the skull through
    a) jugular foramen
    b) hypoglossal canal
    c) foramen magnum
    d) foramen lacerum
1757. Motor supply to the sternocleidomastoid muscle is solely from which of the following nerves?
    a) third and fourth cervical—ventral rami
    b) cranial part of accessory
    c) spinal part of accessory
    d) third and fourth cervical—dorsal rami
1758. Acute torticollis in children is usually because of irritation of which of the following nerves?
    a) vagus
    b) cranial accessory
    c) 3rd & 4th cervical
    d) spinal accessory
1759. Spasmodic torticollis may be relieved by the division/partial excision of which of the following nerves?
    a) hypoglossal
    b) cervical third & fourth
    c) vagus
    d) accessory
1760. The hypoglossal nerve is motor to all muscles of the tongue **except**
    a) palatoglossus
    b) styloglossus
    c) genioglossus
    d) hyoglossus
1761. Which of the following nerves represents the fused ventral roots of probably four cervical nerves?
    a) spinal accessory
    b) hypoglossal
    c) trigeminal
    d) vagus
1762. All of the following nerves lie in series with the ventral nerve roots of the spinal nerves **except**
    a) facial
    b) hypoglossal
    c) oculomotor
    d) trochlear
1763. Which of the following nucleus lies in line with the spinal anterior gray column?
    a) spinal nucleus of trigeminal
    b) hypoglossal
    c) nucleus ambiguus
    d) facial
1764. All of the following cranial nerve nuclei extend into the spinal gray matter **except**
    a) nucleus ambiguus
    b) hypoglossal
    c) spinal nucleus of trigeminal
    d) accessory
1765. Which of the following sulcus of medulla ablongata gives attachment to the rootlets of hypoglossal nerve?
    a) anterior median
    b) posterior median
    c) anterolateral
    d) posterolateral
1766. Which of the following foramen transmits the hypoglossal nerve?
    a) jugular foramen
    b) foramen lacerum
    c) anterior condylar
    d) foramen magnum

1767. Which of the following nerves forms a half spiral turn around the inferior vagal ganglia?
    a) glossopharyngeal   b) spinal part of accessory
    c) cranial part of accessory   d) hypoglossal

1768. Which of the following nerves passes along with vagus nerve between the internal jugular vein and internal carotid artery upto the angle of mandible?
    a) glossopharyngeal   b) hypoglossal
    c) accessory   d) mandibular

1769. Which of the following nerves loops round the inferior sternocleidomastoid branch of the occipital artery?
    a) hypoglossal   b) accessory
    c) lingual   d) glossopharyngeal

1770. Which of the following nerves crosses lateral to both the internal and external carotid arteries?
    a) lingual   b) glossopharyngeal
    c) vagus   d) hypoglossal

1771. The upper root of ansa cervicalis contains the nerve fibres from
    a) the hypoglossal nerve proper   b) first cervical nerve
    c) 2nd & 3rd cervical nerve   d) vagus

1772. All of the following branches of the hypoglossal nerve contain only fibres from the first cervical spinal nerve **except**
    a) muscular to lingual muscles   b) descendens hypoglossi
    c) nerve to thyrohyoid   d) nerve to geniohyoid

1773. The only muscle supplied by the upper root of ansa cervicalis is
    a) superior belly of omohyoid   b) inferior belly of omohyoid
    c) sternohyoid   d) sternothyroid

1774. All of the following muscles are supplied by the ansa cervicalis **except**
    a) thyrohyoid   b) sternohyoid
    c) inferior belly of omohyoid   d) sternothyroid

1775. Complete hypoglossal division will cause
    a) lingual muscle paralysis   b) loss of taste sensation
    c) loss of general sensation of tongue
    d) all of the above

1776. All of the following signs and symptoms are seen with the complete division of the hypoglossal nerve **except**
    a) lingual hemiatrophy   b) loss of taste sensibility
    c) difficulty in swallowing   d) slow articulation

1777. All of the following nerves supply the musculature derived from the cranial myotomes **except**
    a) oculomotor   b) hypoglossal
    c) abducent   d) facial

Chapter IX Head, Face, Neck and Nervous System **175**

1778. All of the following nerves emerge from the brain stem in line with the ventral spinal roots **except**
   a) trochlear b) oculomotor
   c) abducent d) hypoglossal
1779. All of the following nerves innervate derivatives of the branchial arches **except**
   a) trigeminal b) facial
   c) glossopharyngeal d) hypoglossal
1780. Neurons of all of the following ganglia originate partly in ectodermal epibranchial placodes **except**
   a) inferior glossopharyngeal b) trigeminal
   c) inferior vagal d) facial
1781. Neurons of which of the following nerves remain in the epithelial cells of the mucous membrane?
   a) optic b) olfactory
   c) vestibular d) cochlear
1782. Which of the following group of motor nuclei of cranial nerves represent the branchiomotor outflow?
   a) somatic efferent b) general visceral efferent
   c) special visceral efferent d) all of the above
1783. Motor nucleus of which of the following nerves represent the special visceral efferent outflow?
   a) oculomotor b) hypoglossal
   c) abducent d) facial
1784. Motor nuclei of all of the following nerves represent the special visceral efferent column **except**
   a) facial b) glossopharyngeal
   c) hypoglossal d) vagus
1785. Nucleus of which of the following nerves receives largely ipsilateral corticonuclear fibres?
   a) oculomotor b) trochlear c) trigeminal d) facial
1786. All of the following nerves have general visceral effereut nuclei **except**
   a) oculomotor b) facial
   c) glossopharyngeal d) hypoglossal
1787. All of the following nerves carry the special visceral afferent fibres **except**
   a) facial b) glossopharyngeal
   c) vagus d) trigeminal
1788. Which of the following sensory nuclei of trigeminal nerve contains unipolar primary sensory neurons?
   a) mesencephalic b) main sensory
   c) spinal d) all of the above

1789. Dorsal root of the spinal nerves contain
   a) somatic efferent fibres
   b) central processes of neurons of spinal ganglia
   c) peripheral processes of neurons of spinal ganglia
   d) postganglionic sympathetic fibres

1790. Which of the following spinal ganglia usually lie within the dura mater
   a) thoracic
   b) lumbar
   c) sacral
   d) coccygeal

1791. Which of the following spinal ganglia usually lie inside the vertebral canal?
   a) cervical
   b) thoracic
   c) lumbar
   d) sacral

1792. Dorsal roots of cervical spinal nerves have a thickness ratio of three to one to the ventral roots **except**
   a) first cervical
   b) third cervical
   c) fifth cervical
   d) eighth cervical

1793. Ventral rami of which of the following spinal nerves contribute a white ramus communicans to the corresponding sympathetic ganglia?
   a) all
   b) 2nd, 3rd & 4th sacral
   c) all thoracic and first two lumbar
   d) all cervical

1794. Which of the following is the largest spinal nerve?
   a) first thoracic
   b) first lumbar
   c) first sacral
   d) coccygeal

1795. Which of the following is the smallest spinal nerve?
   a) first cervical
   b) first thoracic
   c) first lumbar
   d) coccygeal

1796. Dorsal rami of all of the following spinal nerves do not divide into medial and lateral branches **except**
   a) first cervical
   b) first thoracic
   c) fourth sacral
   d) coccygeal

1797. All of the following cervical spinal dorsal rami supply the skin **except**
   a) first
   b) second
   c) third
   d) fourth

1798. Which of the following cervical spinal dorsal rami supplies the skin?
   a) second
   b) third
   c) fourth
   d) all of the above

1799. Which of the following cervical nerves is known as the suboccipital nerve?
   a) first
   b) second
   c) third
   d) fourth

1800. Which of the following nerve is termed as 'greater occipital nerve'?
   a) medial branch of second cervical dorsal ramus
   b) medial branch of third cervical dorsal ramus
   c) first cervical dorsal ramus
   d) branch of second cervical ventral ramus

1801. Which of the following nerves is the branch of the ventral ramus of second cervical spinal nerve?
   a) greater occipital   b) lesser occipital
   c) suboccipital   d) third occipital

1802. Which of the following nerves ascends with the occipital artery in the scalp?
   a) lesser occipital   b) greater occipital
   c) suboccipital   d) third occipital

1803. All of the following are the ascending superficial branches of the cervical plexus **except**
   a) greater occipital   b) lesser occipital
   c) greater auricular   d) transverse cutaneous

1804. Which of the following nerves is the deep branch of cervical plexus?
   a) phrenic   b) greater auricular
   c) lesser occipital   d) transverse cutaneous

1805. Root value of the phrenic nerve is
   a) C2, C3 & C4   b) C3, C4 & C5
   c) C5, C6 & C7   d) C1, C2 & C3

1806. Which of the following arteries is exclusively cervical in its location?
   a) brachiocephalic   b) right common carotid
   c) left common carotid   d) left subclavian

1807. All of the following are the posterior relations of the thoracic part of left common carotid artery **except**
   a) trachea   b) left recurrent laryngeal nerve
   c) left brachiocephalic vein d) thoracic duct

1808. Common carotid artery divides at the level of
   a) angle of mandible
   b) upper border of cricoid cartilage
   c) upper border of thyroid cartilage
   d) lower border of thyroid cartilage

1809. Which of the tunics of the carotid sinus contains receptor endings of the glossopharyngeal nerve?
   a) intima   b) media
   c) adventitia   d) all of the above

1810. Embedded in the anterior wall of the carotid sheath is the
   a) vagus nerve   b) phrenic nerve
   c) superior root of ansa cervicalis d) sympathetic trunk

1811. All of the following veins cross the common carotid artery **except**
   a) superior thyroid
   b) middle thyroid
   c) inferior thyroid
   d) anterior jugular

1812. All of the following are the posterior relations of the common carotid artery **except**
   a) sympathetic trunk
   b) ascending cervical artery
   c) recurrent laryngeal nerve
   d) inferior thyroid artery

1813. Which of the following structures lies posteriorly between the common carotid artery and the internal jugular vein?
   a) ansa cervicalis
   b) vagus nerve
   c) recurrent laryngeal nerve
   d) sympathetic trunk

1814. Division of common carotid artery corresponds with the intervertebral disc between which of the cervical vertebrae?
   a) second & third
   b) third & fourth
   c) fourth & fifth
   d) fifth & sixth

1815. Which of the following nerves crosses the external carotid artery in the carotid triangle superficially?
   a) hypoglossal
   b) vagus
   c) lingual
   d) ansa cervicalis

1816. All of the following structures separate the internal from the external carotid artery **except**
   a) posterior belly of diagastric
   b) styloid process
   c) glossopharyngeal nerve
   d) part of parotid gland

1817. All of the following arteries are the branches of the external carotid **except**
   a) lingual
   b) ascending pharyngeal
   c) ophthalmic
   d) occipital

1818. Which of the following branches of the external carotid artery accompanies the external laryngeal nerve?
   a) superior thyroid
   b) lingual
   c) facial
   d) ascending pharyngeal

1819. Which of the following laryngeal nerves accompanies the superior laryngeal artery?
   a) internal
   b) external
   c) superior
   d) recurrent

1820. Smallest branch of external carotid artery is
   a) lingual
   b) superior thyroid
   c) facial
   d) ascending pharyngeal

1821. All of the following are the branches of ascending pharyngeal artery **except**
   a) pharyngeal
   b) superior laryngeal
   c) tympanic
   d) meningeal

Chapter IX   Head, Face, Neck and Nervous System   179

1822. Loop of the lingual artery in its first part is crossed by which of the following nerves?
   a) glossopharyngeal
   b) chorda tympani
   c) lingual
   d) hypoglossal
1823. Lingual artery is described into three parts due to its relation to
   a) cornu of hyoid bone
   b) hyoglossus
   c) hypoglossal nerve
   d) middle constrictor
1824. All of the following branches of external carotid artery are crossed superfically by the hypoglossal nerve **except**
   a) lingual
   b) facial
   c) occipital
   d) maxillary
1825. Which of the following branches of the external carotid artery grooves the posterior aspect of the submandibular gland?
   a) lingual
   b) facial
   c) maxillary
   d) ascending pharyngeal
1826. Which of the following nerves accompanies the terminal part of the occipital artery?
   a) greater occipital
   b) lesser occipital
   c) third occipital
   d) greater auricular
1827. Which of the following branches of the external carotid artery reaches the pterygopalatine fossa?
   a) superficial temporal
   b) maxillary
   c) lingual
   d) facial
1828. Which of the following artery passes between the roots of the auriculotemporal nerve?
   a) maxillary
   b) superficial temporal
   c) middle meningeal
   d) deep auricular
1829. Which of the following foramen of skull transmits the accessory meningeal artery?
   a) spinosum
   b) lacerum
   c) rotundum
   d) ovale
1830. Which of the following branches of inferior alveolar artery pierces the sphenomandibular ligament?
   a) lingual
   b) incisor
   c) mental
   d) mylohyoid
1831. Which of the following artery enters the mandibular foramen?
   a) posterior superior alveolar
   b) inferior alveolar
   c) anterior superior alveolar
   d) middle superior alveolar
1832. All of the following are the branches from the first part of the maxillary artery **except**
   a) anterior tympanic
   b) middle meningeal
   c) deep temporal
   d) inferior alveolar

1833. Buccal artery accompanying the buccal nerve is the branch of
   a) inferior alveolar
   b) facial
   c) maxillary
   d) infraorbital

1834. All of the following are the branches of the maxillary artery given in the pterygopalatine fossa **except**
   a) buccal
   b) infraorbital
   c) greater palatine
   d) posterior superior alveolar

1835. Which of the following is the chief extracranial connection between the external and internal carotid arteries?
   a) superior and inferior thyroid arteries
   b) ophthalmic and facial
   c) ophthalmic and infraorbital
   d) ophthalmic and occipital

1836. All of the following are the subdivisions of the anterior triangle of neck **except**
   a) carotid
   b) diagastric
   c) submental
   d) supraclavicular

1837. All of the following muscles form the boundary of the carotid triangle **except**
   a) anterior belly of diagastric
   b) posterior belly of diagastric
   c) sternocleidomastoid
   d) superior belly of omohyoid

1838. All of the following muscles form the floor of the carotid triangle **except**
   a) hyoglossus
   b) thyrohyoid
   c) middle constrictor
   d) superior constrictor

1839. While palpating which of the following triangle of neck, massive arterial pulsation greets the examining fingures?
   a) diagastric
   b) muscular
   c) carotid
   d) submental

1840. Which of the following triangle of neck is unpaired?
   a) muscular
   b) carotid
   c) submental
   d) diagastric

1841. Posterior cervical triangle is divided into two by the
   a) posterior belly of diagastric
   b) anterior scalenus
   c) superior belly of omohyoid
   d) inferior belly of omohyoid

1842. All of the following muscles form the floor of the occipital triangle of neck **except**
   a) longissimus capitis
   b) levator scapulae
   c) scalenus medius
   d) splenius capitis

1843. Which of the following nerve traverses the occipital triangle of neck?
   a) hypoglossal
   b) facial
   c) greater occipital
   d) accessory

Chapter IX — Head, Face, Neck and Nervous System

1844. All of the following nerves cross the occipital triangle **except**
    a) accessory
    b) branches of cervical plexus
    c) upper part of brachial plexus
    d) branches of facial nerve

1845. Brachial plexus is related to the subclavian artery in the supraclavicular triangle
    a) posterosuperiorly
    b) posteriorinferiorly
    c) anterosuperiorly
    d) anteroinferiorly

1846. Which of the following triangles of the neck are is crossed by the external jugular vein?
    a) carotid
    b) supraclavicular
    c) muscular
    d) occipital

1847. All of the following structures lie in the floor of the supraclavicular triangle **except**
    a) first rib
    b) scalenus medius
    c) scalenus posterior
    d) first slip of serratus anterior

1848. Ascending palatine artery is the branch of
    a) facial
    b) lingual
    c) maxillary
    d) ascending pharyngeal

1849. Which of the following part of the internal carotid artery is covered by the lining endothelium?
    a) cervical
    b) petrous
    c) cavernous
    d) cerebral

1850. Which of the following part of the internal carotid artery has no branches?
    a) cervical
    b) petrous
    c) cavernous
    d) cerebral

1851. The ophthalmic artery enters the orbit through the
    a) superior orbital fissure
    b) inferior orbital fissure
    c) foramen rotundum
    d) optic canal

1852. The ophthalmic artery crossess the orbit to the medial wall between the optic nerve and
    a) inferior rectus
    b) superior rectus
    c) superior oblique
    d) inferior oblique

1853. Which of the following branch of the ophthalmic artery may be replaced sometimes by the branch of middle meningeal artery?
    a) lacrimal
    b) central retinal
    c) supraorbital
    d) supratrochlear

1854. Which of the following ciliary arteries form the circumcorneal subconjunctival vascular zone?
    a) anterior
    b) long posterior
    c) short posterior
    d) all of the above

1855. Which of the following parts of the internal carotid artery gives rise to ophthalmic artery?
   a) cervical
   b) petrous
   c) cavernous
   d) cerebral

1856. Which of following arteries gives rise to artery of cerebral haemorrhage?
   a) anterior cerebral
   b) posterior cerebral
   c) middle cerebral
   d) internal carotid

1857. 'Anterior choroidal artery' is the branch of
   a) internal carotid
   b) anterior cerebral
   c) middle cerebral
   d) posterior cerebral

1858. Vein formed by union of posterior division of retromandibular and posterior auricular vein is
   a) common facial
   b) internal jugular
   c) external jugular
   d) maxillary

1859. Inferior bulb of internal jugular vein is located near
   a) its beginning
   b) its termination
   c) its union with common facial vein
   d) its union with external jugular vein

1860. The thoracic duct opens near the union of
   a) right internal jugular with subclavian vein
   b) left internal with external jugular vein
   c) left internal with subclavian vein
   d) right and left brachiocephalic vein

1861. Which of the following nerves may be involved when the superior bulb of internal jugular vein is thrombosed?
   a) glossopharyngeal
   b) vagus
   c) accessory
   d) all of the above

1862. Venous pulsation may be visible in which of the following veins at the root of the neck?
   a) internal jugular
   b) external jugular
   c) anterior jugular
   d) posterior external jugular

1863. Which of the following vein receives the vertebral vein?
   a) external jugular
   b) internal jugular
   c) brachiocephalic
   d) superior vena cava

1864. Vertebral vein emerges out through the foramen tranversarium of which cervical vertebra?
   a) fourth
   b) fifth
   c) sixth
   d) seventh

1865. Diploic veins begin to develop in the cranial bones
   a) during foetal life
   b) at birth
   c) two years after birth
   d) 7 years after birth

Chapter IX   Head, Face, Neck and Nervous System   **183**

1866. Which of the following is the largest diploic vein?
 a) frontal
 b) occipital
 c) anterior temporal
 d) posterior temporal
1867. The basal vein of the cerebrum drains into the
 a) superior sagital sinus
 b) great cerebral vein
 c) internal jugular vein
 d) cavernous sinus
1868. All of the following veins drain into the basal vein **except**
 a) striate veins through anterior perforated substance
 b) anterior cerebral
 c) deep middle cerebral
 d) superior cerebral
1869. Thalamostriate and choroid veins unite to form
 a) internal cerebral vein
 b) straight sinus
 c) basal vein
 d) deep middle cerebral vein
1870. The great cerebral vein terminates into
 a) superior sagittal sinus
 b) striaght sinus
 c) sigmoidal sinus
 d) cavernous sinus
1871. Straight sinus opens in which of the following?
 a) internal jugular vein
 b) occipital sinus
 c) right transverse sinus
 d) left tranverse sinus
1872. Which of the following sinuses is very close to the mastoid antrum and air cells?
 a) transverse
 b) sigmoid
 c) inferior petrosal
 d) occipital
1873. Which of the following muscles of mastication is attached to the coronoid process of mandible?
 a) medial pterygoid
 b) lateral pterygoid
 c) massetter
 d) temporalis
1874. Which of the following muscles of mastication depressess the mandible?
 a) lateral pterygoid
 b) medial pterygoid
 c) massetter
 d) temporalis
1875. All of the following structures are present in the suprasternal space **except**
 a) jugular venous arch
 b) areolar tissue
 c) sternal head of sternocleidomastoid
 d) external jugular vein
1876. Which of the following nerves supplies the anterior belly of digastric muscle?
 a) mandibular
 b) hypoglossal
 c) facial
 d) ansa cervicalis

1877. Which of the following muscles may depress the mandible?
   a) stylohyoid
   b) mylohyoid
   c) geniohyoid
   d) sternohyoid

1878. Which of the following muscles receives the motor nerve supply from the first cervical spinal nerve?
   a) geniohyoid
   b) mylohyoid
   c) anterior belly of digastric
   d) posterior belly of digastric

1879. All of the following muscles elevate the hyoid bone **except**
   a) geniohyoid
   b) stylohyoid
   c) diagastric
   d) omohyoid

1880. Motor supply to all of the following muscles is by ansa cervicalis **except**
   a) sternohyoid
   b) thyrohyoid
   c) geniohyoid
   d) sternothyroid

1881. Which of the following muscles may elevate the larynx?
   a) thyrohyoid
   b) sternohyoid
   c) sternothyroid
   d) superior belly of omohyoid

1882. All of the following muscles are the flexors of head **except**
   a) longus colli
   b) longus capitis
   c) rectus capitis anterior
   d) rectus capitis posterior

1883. Which of the following scalenus muscle is associated with the suprapleural membrane?
   a) anterior
   b) posterior
   c) medius
   d) minimus

1884. All of the following muscles form the boundaries of the suboccipital triangle **except**
   a) rectus capitis major
   b) rectus capitis minor
   c) obliques capitis superior
   d) oblique capitis inferior

1885. Which of the following structures lies in the groove of the posterior atlantal arch?
   a) ventral ramus of c1 nerve
   b) vertebral artery
   c) occipital artery
   d) greater occipital nerve

1886. Nerve supply to all suboccipital muscles is from
   a) greater occipital
   b) third occipital
   c) dorsal ramus of c1
   d) lesser occipital

Chapter X

SPECIAL SENSES

1887. Which of the following bones contain foramen rotundum?
    a) sphenoid   b) temporal
    c) frontal   d) parietal
1888. All of the following bones form the orbit **except**
    a) sphenoid   b) frontal
    c) zygomatic   d) petrous
1889. The roof of the orbit is formed chiefly by which of the following bones?
    a) sphenoid   b) frontal
    c) maxillary   d) zygomatic
1890. The lacrimal fossa is formed by the lacrimal bone and
    a) frontal process of maxillary bone
    b) maxillary process of frontal bone
    c) ethmoid bone   d) nasal bone
1891. The superior orbital fissure is bound above by
    a) greater wing of sphenoid   b) lesser wing of sphenoid
    c) palatine bone   d) ethmoid bone
1892. The optic canal is situated in the
    a) lesser wing of sphenoid   b) greater wing of sphenoid
    c) body of sphenoid   d) none of the above
1893. Which of the following nerves **does not** pass through superior orbital fissure?
    a) abducent   b) nasociliary
    c) trochlear   d) maxillary
1894. Nasolacrimal duct opens into
    a) superior meatus of nose   b) middle meatus of nose
    c) inferior meatus of nose   d) vestibule of mouth
1895. Superior oblique muscle of eyeball is supplied by
    a) trochlear nerve   b) abducent nerve
    c) upper division of oculomotor   d) lower division of oculomotor
1896. Lateral rectus muscle of the eyeball is supplied by
    a) trochlear nerve   b) abducent nerve
    c) oculomotor nerve   d) infraorbital nerve
1897. Sensory nerve supply to the cornea is by
    a) nasociliary nerve   b) lacrimal nerve
    c) supraorbital nerve d) infraorbital nerve

1898. All of the following are the branches of the ophthalmic nerve **except**
 a) frontal
 b) nasociliary
 c) infraorbital
 d) lacrimal

1899. All of the following extraocular muscles are supplied by the oculomotor nerve **except**
 a) medial rectus
 b) lateral rectus
 c) superior rectus
 d) inferior rectus

1900. Which of the following structures is **not** supplied by the lacrimal nerve?
 a) lacrimal gland
 b) lateral part of eyelid
 c) lateral part of conjunctiva
 d) cornea

1901. All of the following structures lie in the lateral wall of cavernous sinus **except**
 a) abducent nerve
 b) trochlear nerve
 c) oculomotor nerve
 d) ophthalmic nerve

1902. Dural sheath of optic nerve gives origin to
 a) medial and lateral rectus
 b) medial and inferior rectus
 c) lateral and superior rectus
 d) lateral and inferior rectus

1903. All of the following are the branches of the ophthalmic artery **except**
 a) central retinal artery
 b) recurrent meningeal artery
 c) lacrimal artery
 d) infraorbital artery

1904. Which of the following **does not** develop from the optic cup?
 a) retina
 b) irideal epithelium
 c) lens
 d) choroid

1905. All of the following arteries supply the optic nerve **except**
 a) central retinal artery
 b) ophthalmic artery
 c) ...rior cerebral artery
 d) infraorbital artery

1906. Which of the following statements is **incorrect** about the optic nerve?
 a) It contains about one million fibres.
 b) Its intracranial length is approximately 10 mm.
 c) It develops from optic stalk.
 d) Its intraocular portion is about 30 mm in length.

1907. Which of the following cranial nerves has the longest intracranial course?
 a) third
 b) fourth
 c) fifth
 d) sixth

1908. In which of the following cranial nerves nucleus lies at the level of inferior colluculus?
 a) third
 b) fourth
 c) fifth
 d) sixth

1909. Which of the following cranial nerves nucleus is associated with the facial colliculus?
 a) third
 b) fourth
 c) fifth
 d) sixth

910. The average thickness of the cornea in the centre is
    a) 0.42 mm b) 0.52 mm
    c) 0.62 mm d) 0.72 mm
911. Which of the following intraocular muscles is supplied by the sympathetic nerve fibres?
    a) ciliary muscle b) sphincter pupillae
    c) dilator pupillae d) none of the above
912. Which of the following layers of the iris is mesodermal in origin?
    a) sphincter pupillae
    b) dilator pupillae
    c) epithelium of posterior layer of iris
    d) stroma of iris
913. Which of the following is neuroectodermal in origin?
    a) sphincter and dilator pupillae muscles
    b) cornea
    c) lens
    d) sclera
914. Axons of which of the following neurons make up the optic nerve?
    a) bipolar neurons b) amacrine neurons
    c) ganglion cells d) horizontal neurons
915. Choriocapillaris originate from
    a) short ciliary arteries b) lacrimal artery
    c) infraorbital artery d) supraorbital artery
916. Which of the following statements regarding the circle of Zinn-Haller is **incorrect**?
    a) It is formed by anastomosis among few short ciliary arteries.
    b) This ring lies in the sclera close to the optic nerve.
    c) It sends branches to the optic disc, optic nerve and the choroid.
    d) It supplies to the cornea.
917. Long posterior ciliary arteries run in the
    a) 9 and 3 O'clock meridian b) 6 and 12 O'clock meridian
    c) 2 and 8 O'clock meridian d) 11 and 5 O'clock meridian
918. Which of the following parts of retina is thickest?
    a) near the optic disc b) near the ora serrata
    c) near the equator d) near the fovea
919. Which part of the ciliary body is derived from neuroectoderm?
    a) muscle b) epithelium
    c) connective tissue stroma d) rossettes
920. The lens of eyeball is derived from
    a) neuroectoderm b) surface ectoderm
    c) mesoderm
    d) neuroectoderm and mesoderm

1921. The permanent vitreous humour is derived from
   a) neuroectoderm
   b) surface ectoderm
   c) mesoderm
   d) surface ectoderm and mesoderm
1922. Which of the following statements regarding the Muller's muscle is **incorrect**?
   a) it arises from posterior pole of eyeball
   b) it is inserted into the superior tarsal plate
   c) it is supplied by sympathetic nerve fibres
   d) it is approximately 15-20 mm wide at its origin.
1923. The human ear is most sensitive to sounds in the range of
   a) 1.5 to 3 Hz
   b) 15 to 30 Hz
   c) 150 to 300 Hz
   d) 1500 to 3000 Hz
1924. In its structure the auricle of ear is a thin plate of
   a) spongy bone
   b) hyaline cartilage
   c) white fibrocartilage
   d) elastic cartilage
1925. All of the following nerves supply sensory innervation to the auricle except
   a) greater occipital
   b) lesser occipital
   c) greater auricular
   d) auriculotemporal
1926. Length of external acoustic meatus in the adult from the floor of the concha is approximately
   a) 0.5 cm
   b) 1.5 cm
   c) 2.5 cm
   d) 3.5 cm
1927. Nerve supply to the posterior and inferior walls of the external auditory meatus is from
   a) auriculotemporal
   b) auricular branch of vagus
   c) greater auricular
   d) lesser occipital
1928. The sinuosity of the external auditory meatus can be straightened to some extent by pulling the auricle
   a) upwards, backwards and laterally
   b) upwards, forwards and laterally
   c) downwards, backwards and laterally
   d) downwards, forwards and laterally
1929. Which of the following walls of the external auditory meatus are longer than the rest?
   a) anterior and inferior
   b) anterior and superior
   c) posterior and inferior
   d) posterior and superior
1930. The tympanic membrane is drawn in at the umbo by the
   a) lateral process of malleus
   b) short process of malleus
   c) handle of malleus
   d) long process of incus

931. The association of earache with toothache is due to involvement of which of the following nerves?
    a) mandibular nerve
    b) maxillary nerve
    c) vagal nerve
    d) greater auricular nerve
932. Surgical incisions of the tympanic membrane should be
    a) posteroinferior
    b) posterosuperior
    c) anterosuperior
    d) anteroinferior
933. The middle ear contains the air derived via the
    a) external auditory meatus
    b) auditory tube
    c) internal auditory meatus
    d) all of the above
934. The least transverse diameter of the tympanic cavity is
    a) opposite the umbo
    b) in the upper part
    c) in the posterior part
    d) in the lower part
935. Which of the following walls of the tympanic cavity is formed by the tegmen tympani?
    a) floor
    b) roof
    c) lateral
    d) medial
936. The tegmen tympani forms the roof of all of the following **except**
    a) internal auditory meatus
    b) tympanic cavity
    c) mastoid antrum
    d) canal for tensor tympani
937. The posterior canaliculus for the chorda tympani nerve is situated in the angle between posterior wall and
    a) medial wall
    b) roof
    c) lateral wall
    d) floor
938. The petrotympanic fissure contains all of the following **except**
    a) tympanic branch of glossopharyngeal nerve
    b) anterior tympanic artery
    c) anterior ligament of the malleus
    d) anterior canaliculus for chorda tympani
939. Most of the circumference of the tympanic membrane is a ring of
    a) bone
    b) fibrocartilage—white
    c) fibrocartilage—elastic
    d) hyaline cartilage
940. Pars flaccida of the tympanic membrane is situated
    a) anteriorly
    b) posteriorly
    c) superiorly
    d) inferiorly
941. Which of the following arteries supply the cuticular stratum of the tympanic membrane?
    a) deep auricular branch of maxillary artery
    b) stylomastoid branch of occipital artery
    c) tympanic branch of maxillary artery
    d) all of the above

1942. Secondary tympanic membrane closes
   a) fenestra vestibuli
   b) fenestra cochlearis
   c) lateral wall of tympanic cavity
   d) opening of auditory tube in the tympanic cavity

1943. All of the following are situated on the posterior wall of the middle ear cavity **except**
   a) promontory
   b) fossa incudius
   c) pyramidal eminence
   d) aditus to mastoid antrum

1944. Which of the following semicircular canal is related to the medial wall of the mastoid antrum?
   a) posterior
   b) lateral
   c) anterior
   d) all of the above

1945. Usual surgical approach to the mastoid antrum is through which of the following wall?
   a) anterior
   b) lateral
   c) posterior
   d) medial

1946. In adults the lateral wall of mastoid antrum corresponds to
   a) supramastoid crest
   b) suprameatal triangle
   c) tip of mastoid process
   d) midpoint of anterior margin of mastoid process

1947. Which of the following air sinus is present at birth?
   a) mastoid antrum
   b) sphenoid
   c) maxillary
   d) frontal

1948. In human skull the mastoid process develops at
   a) birth
   b) the age of two years
   c) at the age of four years
   d) at the age of seven years

1949. Which of the following wall of the tympanic cavity forms the posterior wall of the carotid canal?
   a) anterior
   b) posterior
   c) superior
   d) lateral

1950. The length of the auditory tube in adult human is
   a) 0.36 mm
   b) 3.6 mm
   c) 36 mm
   d) 360 mm

1951. The bony canal above the osseous pharyngotympanic tube is occupied by
   a) stapedius muscle
   b) tensor tympani muscle
   c) anterior ligament of malleus
   d) chorda tympani nerve

1952. Which of the following gives attachment to the tendon of tensor tympani muscle?
   a) handle of malleus
   b) anterior process of malleus
   c) neck of stapes
   d) long process of incus

Chapter X
Special Senses

1953. Which of the following nerve supplies tensor tympani muscle?
   a) auricular branch of vagus
   b) auricular branch of facial
   c) tympanic plexus
   d) branch of the nerve to medial pterygoid

1954. Stapedius muscle is innervated by which of the following nerves?
   a) facial
   b) glossopharyngeal
   c) vagus
   d) mandibular

1955. Which of the following structure is covered by the mucosa of the tympanic cavity?
   a) ossicles
   b) muscles
   c) nerves
   d) all of the above

1956. Which of the following walls of the vestibule of bony labyrinth bears a spherical recess?
   a) medial
   b) lateral
   c) superior
   d) inferior

1957. Upper vestibular area of the lateral end of internal acoustic meatus corresponds with the
   a) utricle
   b) saccule
   c) cochlea
   d) posterior semicircular canal

1958. The foramen singulare in the internal acoustic meatus transmits vestibular nerve fibres to
   a) utricle
   b) saccule
   c) anterior and lateral semicircular canals
   d) posterior semicircular canal

1959. In relation to the vestibule the semicircular canals of the internal ear lie
   a) anterosuperiorly
   b) anteroinferiorly
   c) posterosuperiorly
   d) posteroinferiorly

1960. Number of openings by which semicircular canals open in the vestibule are
   a) 3
   b) 4
   c) 5
   d) 6

1961. The central conical axis of the cochlea is known as the
   a) modiolus
   b) cupola
   c) helicotrema
   d) spiral lamina

1962. Which of the following channels of cochlea is/are blind at cupola?
   a) scala tympani
   b) scala vestibuli
   c) cochlear duct
   d) all of the above

1963. Sensory receptors responsible for audition are located on one of the walls of
   a) scala tympani
   b) scala vestibuli
   c) cochlear duct
   d) all of the above

1964. Which of the following channel of cochlea is separated from the tympanic cavity at the fenestra cochlea?
   a) cochlear duct
   b) scala vestibuli
   c) scala tympani
   d) none of the above

1965. The first turn of osseous cochlear canal underlies the
   a) promontory
   b) arcuate eminence
   c) secondary tympanic membrane
   d) lateral end of internal acoustic meatus

1966. All of the following are the openings in the osseous cochlear canal **except**
   a) cochlear canaliculus
   b) tympanic canaliculus
   c) fenestra cochleae
   d) fenestra vestibuli

1967. Which of the following connects the subarachnoid space to the scala tympani?
   a) tympanic canaliculus
   b) cochlear canaliculus
   c) fenestra cochleae
   d) fenestra vestibuli

1968. All of the following are the parts of the membranous labyrinth of inner ear **except**
   a) cochlear canal
   b) semicircular ducts
   c) saccule
   d) utricle

1969. Which of the following is the part of the osseous labyrinth of inner ear?
   a) utricle
   b) saccule
   c) cochlear duct
   d) semicircular canals

1970. The spiral organ of corti of the inner ear is set on the
   a) spiral lamina
   b) membrana tectoria
   c) vestibular membrane
   d) basilar membrane

1971. Stria vascularis of the cochlear duct of the inner ear is present on the
   a) basilar membrane
   b) vestibular membrane
   c) lateral wall of the duct
   d) membrana tectoria

1972. The tunnel of corti lies between the
   a) inner and outer rod cells
   b) spiral lamina and inner rod cells
   c) outer rod cells and the spiral prominence
   d) vestibular membrane and the membrana tectoria

1973. Which of the following parts of the cochlear duct of the inner ear is gelationous proteinaceous material?
   a) membrana tectoria
   b) stria vascularis
   c) vestibular membrane
   d) basilar membrane

Chapter X
Special Senses

1974. Which of the following cells of the spiral organ of corti bear the stereociila?
   a) phalangeal cells
   b) hair cells
   c) rod cells
   d) all of the above

1975. The vestibular ganglia of the vestibulocochlear nerve lies
   a) on the spiral lamina or the cochlea
   b) in the spherical recess of osseous labyrinth
   c) on the trunk of the nerve in the internal acoustic meatus
   d) on the macula of the utricle and saccule

1976. Taste buds are most numerous in which papillae of the tongue?
   a) filliform
   b) circumvallate
   c) fungiform
   d) foliate

1977. Taste buds are not seen in which of the following region of the tongue?
   a) tip
   b) margins
   c) central part of dorsum
   d) postorior third of tongue

1978. Gustatory nerve fibres are the peripheral processes of the unipolar neurons in all of the following ganglia **except**
   a) geniculate
   b) trigeminal
   c) inferior glossopharyngeal
   d) inferior vagal

1979. Tractus solitarius is formed by central processes of neurons in all of the following ganglia **except**
   a) trigeminal
   b) facial
   c) inferior vagal
   d) inferior glossopharyngeal

1980. Secondary gustarory fibres terminate in which of the following thalamic nucleus?
   a) ventralis posterior medialis (VPM)
   b) ventralis posterior lateralis (VPL)
   c) ventralis anterior
   d) medialis dorsalis

1981. Which of the following is the gustatory cortical area?
   a) anteroinferior part of postcentral cortex
   b) lips of calcarine sulcus
   c) superior temporal gyrus
   d) cingulate gyrus

1982. The oral part of tongue is derived from which of the following branchial arches?
   a) first
   b) second
   c) third
   d) all of the above

1983. All of the following parts of the nasal cavity constitute the olfactory region **except**
   a) the floor
   b) the roof
   c) upper part of nasal septum
   d) superior concha

1984. Which of the following regions of the nasal cavity bear coarse hairs?
   a) the vestibular
   b) olfactory
   c) respiratory
   d) all of the above

1985. Above the superior nasal concha a triangular recess bears the opening of which of the air sinuses?
   a) sphenoidal
   b) maxillary
   c) frontal
   d) anterior ethmoidal

1986. Which of the following meatus bears the openings of the posterior ethmoidal air sinuses?
   a) superior
   b) middle
   c) inferior
   d) all of the above

1987. Which of the meatuses of the lateral nasal wall bears the bulla ethmoidalis?
   a) supreme
   b) superior
   c) middle
   d) inferior

1988. Bulging of which of the following air sinuses produce the bulla ethmoidalis on the lateral nasal wall?
   a) maxillary
   b) anterior ethmoidal
   c) posterior ethmoidal
   d) middle ethmoidal

1989. The anterior ethmoidal air sinus opens
   a) on the bulla ethmoidalis
   b) in the ethmoidal infundibulum
   c) below the bulla ethmoidalis
   d) above the bulla ethmoidalis

1990. All of the following air sinuses open in the middle meatus of lateral nasal wall **except**
   a) frontal
   b) sphenoidal
   c) anterior ethmoidal
   d) maxillary

1991. Which of the following meatuses of lateral nasal wall bear the opening of nasolacrimal duct?
   a) supreme
   b) superior
   c) middle
   d) inferior

1992. What type of neurons the olfactory receptor cells are?
   a) unipolar
   b) pseudounipolar
   c) bipolar
   d) multipolar

1993. Which of the following receptor cells are the primary sensory neurons?
   a) auditory
   b) vestibular
   c) gustatory
   d) olfactory

1994. The peripheral processes of the olfactory receptor cells bear
   a) cilia
   b) stereocilia
   c) microvilli
   d) none of the above

Chapter X   Special Senses   195

1995. The ability to regenerate primary sensory neurons is unique in which of the following sensory apparatus in mammals?
   a) visual
   b) gustatory
   c) auditory
   d) olfactory

1996. Lymphatic drainage of which of the following air sinuses is to the retropharyngeal nodes?
   a) sphenoidal
   b) anterior ethmoidal
   c) frontal
   d) maxillary

1997. Lymphatic drainage of all of the following air sinuses is to the submandibular lymph nodes **except**
   a) frontal
   b) maxillary
   c) sphenoidal & posterior ethmoidal
   d) anterior & middle ethmoidal

1998. Opening of which of the following paranasal sinuses is high above its floor?
   a) frontal
   b) sphenoidal
   c) posterior ethmoidal
   d) maxillary

Chapter XI

RADIOLOGY AND IMAGING METHODS

1999. What kind of waves X-rays are?
   a) electric
   b) electromagnetic
   c) magnetic
   d) sound

2000. X-rays were discovered in 1895 by
   a) Wilhelm Konrad Roentgen
   b) Howard Sochurek
   c) Brian S. Worthington
   d) None of the above

2001. All of the following are the properties of X-rays **except**
   a) they show penetrating power
   b) when they strike a photosensitive film, the film gets photosensitized
   c) X-rays cause the metallic salts to fluoresce
   d) X-rays bounce back towards the source

2002. Which of the following properties of X-rays is considered to be potentially dangerous in diagnostic procedures?
   a) penetrating power
   b) photographic effect
   c) fluorescent effect
   d) biological effect

2003. Which of the following properties of X-rays is beneficial for therapeutic purpose?
   a) penetrating power
   b) photographic effect
   c) fluorescent effect
   d) biological effect

2004. Which of the following statements regarding X-rays is **incorrect**?
   a) plain X-rays are useful to study bones
   b) X-rays can destroy normal cells more easily than abnormal cells
   c) X-rays are used in the treatment of various cancers
   d) repeated exposure to X-rays can cause genetic mutations.

2005. All of the following terms can be used to describe an X-ray image **except**
   a) sonograph
   b) skiagram
   c) radiograph
   d) roentgenogram

2006. Which of the following will produce black shadow on the negative X-rays film?
   a) bone
   b) soft tissues
   c) skin
   d) gas

2007. Which of the following will produce most radiopaque shadow on the X-ray film?
   a) bone
   b) enamel of teeth
   c) muscles
   d) gas

Chapter XI — Radiology and Imaging Methods

2008. Radiography is based on
 a) differential absorption of X-rays by different tissues
 b) equal absorption of X-rays by different tissues
 c) obstruction of X-rays by all the tissues
 d) none of the above

2009. Degree of absorption of X-rays depends on
 a) weight of the matter
 b) density of the matter
 c) size of the structure
 d) none of the above

2010. Structures which are easily penetrated by X-rays are described as
 a) translucent
 b) radiolucent
 c) radioopaque
 d) transopaque

2011. View of X-rays indicates
 a) surface of the X-ray film seen
 b) surface of the body part-seen on the film
 c) the direction of flow of X-rays
 d) none of the above

2012. In posteroanterior radiographic (PA) view
 a) X-rays pass from anterior to posterior surface
 b) X-rays pass from posterior to anterior surface
 c) posterior surface faces the X-ray plate
 d) anterior surface faces the X-ray tube

2013. The part of the body facing the X-rays plate casts a shadow
 a) sharper than the part facing the X-ray tube
 b) less sharper than the part facing the X-ray tube
 c) equal in sharpness to that of the part facing the X-ray tube
 d) not clearly seen on X-ray film

2014. The chest X-rays are usually taken in
 a) AP view
 b) PA view
 c) oblique view
 d) lateral view

2015. Plain radiography is **not** useful to study
 a) hallow viscera
 b) bones
 c) lungs
 d) paranasal air sinuses

2016. All of the following statements regarding the contrast radiography **are correct except**
 a) it is done after artificial accentuation of the contrast
 b) radioopaque media are used to fill the cavities of hollow viscera
 c) radiolucent media can be used to fill the cavities of hollow viscera
 d) bones can well be studied by contrast radiography

2017. Which of the following is the radiopaque contrast medium?
 a) air
 b) oxygen
 c) carbon dioxide
 d) iodine compounds

2018. All of the following are the radioopaque media **except**
 a) barium sulphate solution
 b) iodine compound
 c) iodized oils
 d) nitrogen

2019. Which of the following provides images comparable to anatomical slices
 a) skiagrams
 b) CT scans
 c) sonography
 d) none of the above

2020. Which of the following provides three dimensional radiography?
 a) holography
 b) xeroradiography
 c) CT scans
 d) skiagrams

2021. Xeroradiography provides better images of
 a) soft tissues
 b) bones
 c) gases
 d) fluids

2022. Which of the following scanning procedures uses the high frequency sound waves?
 a) CT scanning
 b) MRI
 c) contrast radiography
 d) ultrasonography

2023. The sound waves used for ultrasonography are
 a) below the range of hearing
 b) within the range of human hearing
 c) above the range of human hearing
 d) all of the above

2024. Which of the following scanning procedures is safe in obsteric problems?
 a) CT scan
 b) X-rays
 c) sonography
 d) MRI

2025. Which of the following procedures convert X-ray pictures into digital computer code to make high resolution video images?
 a) CT scan
 b) MRI
 c) sonography
 d) none

2026. In which of the following techniques teeth and bones cannot be observed?
 a) CT scan
 b) MRI
 c) sonography
 d) none

2027. Which of the following technique reflects only water in the body?
 a) CT scan
 b) MRI
 c) sonography
 d) none

2028. Which of the following images reverts the varying densities of hydrogen atoms and their interaction with surrounding tissues in a cross section of body?
 a) MRI
 b) CT scan
 c) sonography
 d) none of the above

2029. Which of the following is a very effective means of examining the spinal cord?
   a) MRI
   b) CT scan
   c) sonography
   d) contrast radiography

2030. The only body scanning technique recommended for pregnant women is
   a) CT scan
   b) MRI
   c) sonography
   d) X-rays

2031. Routine chest X-ray films are ordinarily made in the erect position for which of the conditions?
   a) renal failure
   b) urinary bladder stone
   c) obstruction of urethra
   d) colon obstruction

2032. Which of the following radiographic procedure is recommended to detect the fallopian tube obstruction?
   a) intravenous pyelography
   b) salphingography
   c) barium enema
   d) KUB

2033. The method of choice in preliminary evaluation of biliary obstruction is
   a) ultrasonography
   b) oral cholecystography
   c) CT scan
   d) intravenous cholangiography

2034. Which of the following procedures can be performed without preparation of a patient?
   a) KUB
   b) barium enema
   c) barium meal
   d) cholecystography

2035. Carotid angiography is indicated in
   a) ant. cerebral artery aneurysm
   b) skull fracture
   c) chronic sinusitis
   d) internal hydrocephalus

2036. Which is the preferred screen-imaging modality for neonatal renal problem?
   a) intravenous pyelography
   b) CT scan
   c) ultrasonography
   d) radionucleide imaging

ANSWERS

CHAPTER II : EMBRYOLOGY

1. (b)	2. (c)	3. (b)	4. (a)	5. (a)	6. (d)
7. (b)	8. (a)	9. (a)	10. (a)	11. (c)	12. (b)
13. (d)	14. (c)	15. (b)	16. (b)	17. (c)	18. (d)
19. (a)	20. (c)	21. (d)	22. (c)	23. (d)	24. (b)
25. (c)	26. (d)	27. (a)	28. (c)	29. (d)	30. (b)
31. (c)	32. (a)	33. (d)	34. (a)	35. (d)	36. (c)
37. (d)	38. (a)	39. (c)	40. (a)	41. (d)	42. (a)
43. (b)	44. (c)	45. (a)	46. (b)	47. (a)	48. (a)
49. (d)	50. (a)	51. (b)	52. (c)	53. (b)	54. (a)
55. (c)	56. (d)	57. (b)	58. (c)	59. (b)	60. (a)
61. (c)	62. (c)	63. (b)	64. (a)	65. (b)	66. (c)
67. (c)	68. (a)	69. (a)	70. (b)	71. (b)	72. (b)
73. (c)	74. (a)	75. (c)	76. (c)	77. (b)	78. (c)
79. (b)	80. (c)	81. (d)	82. (a)	83. (b)	84. (c)
85. (a)	86. (d)	87. (b)	88. (a)	89. (c)	90. (a)
91. (a)	92. (a)	93. (c)	94. (c)	95. (b)	96. (d)
97. (b)	98. (a)	99. (b)	100. (c)	101. (b)	102. (a)
103. (c)	104. (d)	105. (a)	106. (a)	107. (d)	108. (c)
109. (a)	110. (a)	111. (b)	112. (d)	113. (a)	114. (d)
115. (d)	116. (c)	117. (d)	118. (d)	119. (a)	120. (b)
121. (d)	122. (b)	123. (b)	124. (c)	125. (c)	126. (a)
127. (c)	128. (a)	129. (a)	130. (c)	131. (d)	132. (c)
133. (a)	134. (a)	135. (b)	136. (c)	137. (a)	138. (a)
139. (d)	140. (a)	141. (c)	142. (d)	143. (a)	144. (a)
145. (c)	146. (b)	147. (b)	148. (c)	149. (d)	150. (c)
151. (a)	152. (a)	153. (c)	154. (c)	155. (c)	156. (d)
157. (b)	158. (c)	159. (d)	160. (b)	161. (a)	162. (b)
163. (c)	164. (c)	165. (a)	166. (c)	167. (c)	168. (b)
169. (d)	170. (c)	171. (b)	172. (a)	173. (c)	174. (b)
175. (d)	176. (b)	177. (c)	178. (b)	179. (c)	180. (a)
181. (d)	182. (b)	183. (c)	184. (c)	185. (c)	186. (a)

187. (a)	188. (a)	189. (b)	190. (d)	191. (c)	192. (a)	
193. (c)	194. (a)	195. (d)	196. (b)	197. (a)	198. (b)	
199. (c)	200. (a)	201. (c)	202. (b)	203. (b)	204. (a)	
205. (d)	206. (b)	207. (a)	208. (a)	209. (d)	210. (c)	
211. (b)	212. (d)	213. (b)	214. (a)	215. (b)	216. (c)	
217. (d)	218. (a)	219. (c)	220. (b)	221. (a)	222. (b)	
223. (b)	224. (a)	225. (d)	226. (a)	227. (a)	228. (d)	
229. (b)	230. (a)	231. (c)	232. (c)	233. (b)	234. (c)	
235. (a)	236. (c)	237. (a)	238. (b)	239. (a)	240. (d)	
241. (b)	242. (c)	243. (d)	244. (b)	245. (d)	246. (c)	
247. (d)	248. (a)	249. (c)	250. (b)	251. (b)	252. (b)	
253. (b)	254. (c)	255. (c)	256. (d)			

CHAPTER III : GENETICS

257. (b)	258. (d)	259. (b)	260. (a)	261. (c)	262. (d)	
263. (b)	264. (d)	265. (a)	266. (a)	267. (d)	268. (b)	
269. (c)	270. (d)	271. (c)	272. (d)	273. (b)	274. (c)	
275. (b)	276. (b)	277. (c)	278. (c)	279. (b)	280. (c)	
281. (c)	282. (c)	283. (b)	284. (a)	285. (b)	286. (c)	
287. (d)	288. (b)	289. (b)	290. (b)	291. (d)	292. (d)	
293. (c)	294. (d)	295. (d)	296. (a)	297. (b)	298. (a)	
299. (c)	300. (b)	301. (b)	302. (a)	303. (b)	304. (a)	
305. (b)	306. (c)	307. (b)	308. (c)	309. (c)	310. (b)	
311. (a)	312. (c)	313. (b)	314. (c)	315. (b)	316. (b)	
317. (c)	318. (d)	319. (d)	320. (d)	321. (b)	322. (c)	
323. (d)	324. (d)	325. (c)	326. (c)	327. (c)	328. (b)	
329. (d)	330. (d)	331. (c)	332. (b)	333. (b)		

CHAPTER IV : GENERAL ANATOMY

334. (b)	335. (c)	336. (d)	337. (a)	338. (b)	339. (a)	
340. (c)	341. (d)	342. (d)	343. (b)	344. (c)	345. (c)	
346. (d)	347. (c)	348. (a)	349. (d)	350. (c)	351. (b)	
352. (c)	353. (a)	354. (d)	355. (c)	356. (d)	357. (b)	
358. (a)	359. (d)	360. (d)	361. (b)	362. (c)	363. (d)	
364. (d)	365. (b)	366. (b)	367. (b)	368. (d)	369. (d)	
370. (c)	371. (a)	372. (c)	373. (d)	374. (d)	375. (d)	

376. (d)	377. (a)	378. (c)	379. (b)	380. (c)	381. **(d)**
382. (d)	383. (c)	384. (c)	385. (b)	386. (b)	387. **(b)**
388. (a)	389. (d)	390. (b)	391. (b)	392. (d)	393. (b)
394. (d)	395. (b)	396. (c)	397. (c)	398. (d)	399. **(a)**
400. (d)	401. (b)	402. (b)	403. (c)	404. (b)	405. **(b)**
406. (a)	407. (b)	408. (a)	409. (d)	410. (b)	411. **(b)**
412. (b)	413. (a)	414. (b)	415. (c)	416. (d)	417. **(c)**
418. (c)	419. (c)	420. (b)	421. (c)	422. (b)	423. **(c)**
424. (a)	425. (a)	426. (d)	427. (a)	428. (b)	429. **(a)**
430. (a)	431. (b)	432. (c)	433. (b)	434. (d)	435. **(a)**
436. (a)	437. (b)	438. (d)	439. (b)	440. (b)	441. **(b)**
442. (c)	443. (d)	444. (a)	445. (d)	446. (b)	447. (a)
448. (c)	449. (d)	450. (c)	451. (a)	452. (b)	453. (d)
454. (b)	455. (a)	456. (a)	457. (d)	458. (b)	459. (b)
460. (a)	461. (a)	462. (a)	463. (b)	464. (a)	465. **(b)**
466. (d)	467. (a)	468. (c)	469. (c)	470. (d)	471. **(a)**
472. (a)	473. (a)	474. (b)	475. (c)	476. (c)	477. **(a)**
478. (b)	479. (b)	480. (a)	481. (c)	482. (d)	483. **(c)**
484. (d)	485. (a)	486. (a)	487. (a)	488. (c)	489. **(a)**
490. (d)	491. (b)	492. (c)	493. (b)	494. (b)	495. (b)
496. (c)	497. (c)	498. (a)	499. (c)	500. (b)	501. (a)
502. (b)	503. (c)	504. (c)	505. (b)	506. (d)	507. (c)
508. (b)					

CHAPTER V : UPPER LIMB

509. (d)	510. (b)	511. (c)	512. (b)	513. (a)	514. (b)
515. (a)	516. (d)	517. (c)	518. (d)	519. (b)	520. (b)
521. (d)	522. (c)	523. (a)	524. (c)	525. (d)	526. **(b)**
527. (a)	528. (b)	529. (c)	530. (c)	531. (a)	532. (c)
533. (a)	534. (c)	535. (b)	536. (c)	537. (b)	538. (b)
539. (c)	540. (a)	541. (c)	542. (d)	543. (c)	544. (b)
545. (a)	546. (c)	547. (a)	548. (d)	549. (a)	550. **(c)**
551. (a)	552. (b)	553. (a)	554. (a)	555. (c)	556. **(a)**
557. (d)	558. (a)	559. (d)	560. (a)	561. (a)	562. **(a)**
563. (b)	564. (a)	565. (a)	566. (a)	567. (a)	568. **(a)**
569. (c)	570. (c)	571. (a)	572. (d)	573. (b)	574. **(d)**
575. (b)	576. (d)	577. (d)	578. (a)	579. (d)	580. **(d)**

581. (c) 582. (a) 583. (d) 584. (c) 585. (a) 586. (b)
587. (a) 588. (b) 589. (c) 590. (d) 591. (c) 592. (c)
593. (d) 594. (b) 595. (d) 596. (b) 597. (a) 598. (d)
599. (a) 600. (b) 601. (c) 602. (d) 603. (c) 604. (a)
605. (d) 606. (b) 607. (b) 608. (d) 609. (b) 610. (c)
611. (a) 612. (c) 613. (d) 614. (d) 615. (c) 616. (d)
617. (d) 618. (c) 619. (d) 620. (c) 621. (d) 622. (c)
623. (c) 624. (b) 625. (b) 626. (a) 627. (b) 628. (b)
629. (b) 630. (d) 631. (b) 632. (c) 633. (a) 634. (d)
635. (a) 636. (c) 637. (b) 638. (c) 639. (a) 640. (d)
641. (c) 642. (c) 643. (d) 644. (b) 645. (a) 646. (c)
647. (b) 648. (b) 649. (d) 650. (b) 651. (a) 652. (b)
653. (c) 654. (c) 655. (d) 656. (b) 657. (a) 658. (c)
659. (d) 660. (a) 661. (c) 662. (a) 663. (b) 664. (b)
665. (c) 666. (b) 667. (d) 668. (b) 669. (a) 670. (b)
671. (c) 672. (d) 673. (a) 674. (b) 675. (a) 676. (d)
677. (a) 678. (d) 679. (d) 680. (b) 681. (b) 682. (a)
683. (b) 684. (c) 685. (d) 686. (a) 687. (a) 688. (a)
689. (b) 690. (a) 691. (b) 692. (b) 693. (d) 694. (c)
695. (d) 696. (c) 697. (a) 698. (d) 699. (d) 700. (a)
701. (c) 702. (b) 703. (d) 704. (c) 705. (d) 706. (c)
707. (b) 708. (d) 709. (c) 710. (b) 711. (a) 712. (d)
713. (d) 714. (d) 715. (c) 716. (c)

CHAPTER VI : LOWER LIMB

717. (b) 718. (d) 719. (b) 720. (b) 721. (d) 722. (b)
723. (b) 724. (b) 725. (d) 726. (a) 727. (b) 728. (b)
729. (c) 730. (a) 731. (d) 732. (c) 733. (b) 734. (b)
735. (a) 736. (d) 737. (a) 738. (b) 739. (d) 740. (c)
741. (b) 742. (a) 743. (a) 744. (d) 745. (c) 746. (a)
747. (a) 748. (b) 749. (c) 750. (a) 751. (d) 752. (c)
753. (c) 754. (b) 755. (c) 756. (d) 757. (b) 758. (c)
759. (b) 760. (a) 761. (a) 762. (c) 763. (b) 764. (c)
765. (b) 766. (b) 767. (d) 768. (c) 769. (c) 770. (d)
771. (a) 772. (b) 773. (c) 774. (d) 775. (a) 776. (c)
777. (b) 778. (a) 779. (d) 780. (b) 781. (c) 782. (a)
783. (d) 784. (c) 785. (a) 786. (d) 787. (b) 788. (a)

789. (c)	790. (b)	791. (a)	792. (a)	793. (b)	794. (d)
795. (b)	796. (a)	797. (c)	798. (d)	799. (d)	800. (c)
801. (b)	802. (a)	803. (c)	804. (b)	805. (a)	806. (b)
807. (c)	808. (d)	809. (b)	810. (a)	811. (c)	812. (a)
813. (b)	814. (c)	815. (b)	816. (a)	817. (d)	818. (d)
819. (b)	820. (d)	821. (d)	822. (d)	823. (d)	824. (a)
825. (b)	826. (a)	827. (b)	828. (b)	829. (c)	830. (c)
831. (b)	832. (d)	833. (d)	834. (a)	835. (c)	836. (b)
837. (a)	838. (a)	839. (b)	840. (c)	841. (b)	842. (a)
843. (b)	844. (c)	845. (c)	846. (d)	847. (c)	848. (c)
849. (b)	850. (c)	851. (a)	852. (d)	853. (c)	854. (d)
855. (b)	856. (a)	857. (a)	858. (b)	859. (c)	860. (c)
861. (a)	862. (c)	863. (c)	864. (b)	865. (b)	866. (a)
867. (a)	868. (c)	869. (d)	870. (d)	871. (b)	872. (b)
873. (b)	874. (c)	875. (c)	876. (b)	877. (d)	878. (d)
879. (a)	880. (b)	881. (a)	882. (d)	883. (d)	884. (a)
885. (d)	886. (a)	887. (d)	888. (d)	889. (d)	890. (d)
891. (c)	892. (b)	893. (a)	894. (c)	895. (a)	896. (d)
897. (c)	898. (b)	899. (c)	900. (b)	901. (a)	902. (a)
903. (b)	904. (a)	905. (a)	906. (b)	907. (c)	908. (c)
909. (b)	910. (c)	911. (b)	912. (b)	913. (d)	914. (a)
915. (b)	916. (a)	917. (a)	918. (a)	919. (d)	920. (c)
921. (b)	922. (a)	923. (b)	924. (d)	925. (c)	926. (a)
927. (b)	928. (a)	929. (c)	930. (a)	931. (c)	932. (b)
933. (c)	934. (c)	935. (a)	936. (c)	937. (d)	938. (d)
939. (c)	940. (c)	941. (a)	942. (b)	943. (b)	944. (c)
945. (c)	946. (c)	947. (d)	948. (a)	949. (c)	950. (b)
951. (c)	952. (a)	953. (c)	954. (b)	955. (a)	956. (b)
957. (d)	958. (b)	959. (b)	960. (a)	961. (c)	962. (d)
963. (c)	964. (a)	965. (c)	966. (b)	967. (c)	968. (c)
969. (b)	970. (a)	971. (d)	972. (d)	973. (b)	974. (b)
975. (b)	976. (d)	977. (a)	978. (c)	979. (d)	980. (c)
981. (a)	982. (d)	983. (a)			

CHAPTER VII : THORAX

984. (d)	985. (a)	986. (d)	987. (c)	988. (a)	989. (a)
990. (d)	991. (b)	992. (d)	993. (b)	994. (d)	995. (c)

996. (d)   997. (b)   998. (c)   999. (b)   1000. (a)   1001. (c)
1002. (c) 1003. (d) 1004. (b) 1005. (c) 1006. (d)   1007. (a)
1008. (b) 1009. (b)

CHAPTER VIII : ABDOMEN, PELVIS AND PERINEUM

1010. (d) 1011. (c) 1012. (d) 1013. (b) 1014. (d) 1015. (c)
1016. (c) 1017. (b) 1018. (d) 1019. (c) 1020. (a) 1021. (c)
1022. (d) 1023. (c) 1024. (b) 1025. (b) 1026. (c) 1027. (b)
1028. (c) 1029. (c) 1030. (b) 1031. (a) 1032. (d) 1033. (c)
1034. (a) 1035. (a) 1036. (b) 1037. (c) 1038. (c) 1039. (b)
1040. (b) 1041. (d) 1042. (c) 1043. (a) 1044. (a) 1045. (b)
1046. (b) 1047. (b) 1048. (b) 1049. (c) 1050. (b) 1051. (a)
1052. (c) 1053. (c) 1054. (c) 1055. (b) 1056. (c) 1057. (c)
1058. (a) 1059. (d) 1060. (c) 1061. (b) 1062. (b) 1063. (c)
1064. (a) 1065. (a) 1066. (b) 1067. (a) 1068. (b) 1069. (a)
1070. (b) 1071. (d) 1072. (a) 1073. (a) 1074. (d) 1075. (d)
1076. (a) 1077. (d) 1078. (a) 1079. (c) 1080. (a) 1081. (a)
1082. (b) 1083. (b) 1084. (a) 1085. (c) 1086. (d) 1087. (b)
1088. (d) 1089. (d) 1090. (a) 1091. (b) 1092. (d) 1093. (a)
1094. (a) 1095. (c) 1096. (a) 1097. (a) 1098. (d) 1099. (a)
1100. (d) 1101. (a) 1102. (a) 1103. (a) 1104. (c) 1105. (b)
1106. (c) 1107. (b) 1108. (b) 1109. (b) 1110. (c) 1111. (c)
1112. (c) 1113. (a) 1114. (a) 1115. (d) 1116. (a) 1117. (a)
1118. (c) 1119. (c) 1120. (d) 1121. (d) 1122. (b) 1123. (a)
1124. (b) 1125. (a) 1126. (a) 1127. (c) 1128. (d) 1129. (c)
1130. (c) 1131. (b) 1132. (c) 1133. (c) 1134. (b) 1135. (d)
1136. (c) 1137. (d) 1138. (c) 1139. (b) 1140. (c) 1141. (a)
1142. (a) 1143. (b) 1144. (c) 1145. (b) 1146. (d) 1147. (a)
1148. (b) 1149. (b) 1150. (b) 1151. (c) 1152. (d) 1153. (c)
1154. (c) 1155. (d) 1156. (b) 1157. (a) 1158. (b) 1159. (d)
1160. (b) 1161. (a) 1162. (a) 1163. (c) 1164. (c) 1165. (c)
1166. (d) 1167. (d) 1168. (c) 1169. (b) 1170. (d) 1171. (b)
1172. (c) 1173. (d) 1174. (c) 1175. (b) 1176. (b) 1177. (a)
1178. (d) 1179. (a) 1180. (b) 1181. (b) 1182. (d) 1183. (c)
1184. (d) 1185. (c) 1186. (a) 1187. (a) 1188. (a) 1189. (d)
1190. (b) 1191. (d) 1192. (b) 1193. (c) 1194. (b) 1195. (a)
1196. (c) 1197. (d) 1198. (b) 1199. (b) 1200. (a) 1201. (b)

Answers 207

1202. (c)	1203. (b)	1204. (d)	1205. (a)	1206. (d)	1207. (a)	
1208. (d)	1209. (b)	1210. (a)	1211. (c)	1212. (c)	1213. (a)	
1214. (d)	1215. (b)	1216. (d)	1217. (d)	1218. (a)	1219. (c)	
1220. (a)	1221. (b)	1222. (b)	1223. (d)	1224. (a)	1225. (a)	
1226. (a)	1227. (a)	1228. (a)	1229. (b)	1230. (c)	1231. (b)	
1232. (a)	1233. (b)	1234. (a)	1235. (b)	1236. (c)	1237. (d)	
1238. (b)	1239. (b)	1240. (d)	1241. (b)	1242. (d)	1243. (a)	
1244. (b)	1245. (a)	1246. (d)	1247. (b)	1248. (a)	1249. (a)	
1250. (a)	1251. (c)	1252. (b)	1253. (b)	1254. (b)	1255. (b)	
1256. (c)	1257. (a)	1258. (d)	1259. (b)	1260. (d)	1261. (c)	
1262. (a)	1263. (a)	1264. (a)	1265. (b)	1266. (c)	1267. (d)	
1268. (b)	1269. (c)	1270. (b)	1271. (a)	1272. (a)	1273. (c)	
1274. (c)	1275. (a)	1276. (c)	1277. (d)	1278. (c)	1279. (a)	
1280. (d)	1281. (c)	1282. (b)	1283. (b)	1284. (c)	1285. (a)	
1286. (b)	1287. (c)	1288. (a)	1289. (a)	1290. (d)	1291. (c)	
1292. (a)	1293. (b)	1294. (a)	1295. (c)	1296. (d)	1297. (a)	
1298. (c)	1299. (d)	1300. (d)	1301. (c)	1302. (c)	1303. (a)	
1304. (a)	1305. (b)	1306. (c)	1307. (c)	1308. (a)	1309. (d)	
1310. (d)	1311. (b)	1312. (b)	1313. (d)	1314. (b)	1315. (b)	
1316. (d)	1317. (c)	1318. (c)	1319. (b)	1320. (d)	1321. (b)	
1322. (b)	1323. (a)	1324. (b)	1325. (c)	1326. (b)		

CHAPTER IX : HEAD, FACE, NECK AND NERVOUS SYSTEM

1327. (d)	1328. (c)	1329. (d)	1330. (c)	1331. (b)	1332. (c)
1333. (c)	1334. (c)	1335. (a)	1336. (b)	1337. (c)	1338. (c)
1339. (d)	1340. (d)	1341. (d)	1342. (c)	1343. (b)	1344. (d)
1345. (c)	1346. (a)	1347. (a)	1348. (a)	1349. (d)	1350. (c)
1351. (c)	1352. (a)	1353. (c)	1354. (c)	1355. (a)	1356. (b)
1357. (c)	1358. (b)	1359. (a)	1360. (c)	1361. (b)	1362. (b)
1363. (b)	1364. (b)	1365. (d)	1366. (a)	1367. (d)	1368. (b)
1369. (a)	1370. (c)	1371. (b)	1372. (a)	1373. (a)	1374. (b)
1375. (d)	1376. (a)	1377. (b)	1378. (d)	1379. (b)	1380. (c)
1381. (c)	1382. (b)	1383. (c)	1384. (c)	1385. (d)	1386. (a)
1387. (c)	1388. (a)	1389. (c)	1390. (b)	1391. (c)	1392. (a)
1393. (c)	1394. (b)	1395. (d)	1396. (c)	1397. (b)	1398. (a)
1399. (d)	1400. (d)	1401. (c)	1402. (b)	1403. (b)	1404. (d)

1405. (a)	1406. (c)	1407. (d)	1408. (c)	1409. (b)	1410. (c)
1411. (a)	1412. (b)	1413. (d)	1414. (a)	1415. (d)	1416. (c)
1417. (c)	1418. (c)	1419. (d)	1420. (a)	1421. (d)	1422. (d)
1423. (b)	1424. (a)	1425. (b)	1426. (b)	1427. (b)	1428. (b)
1429. (b)	1430. (c)	1431. (d)	1432. (d)	1433. (b)	1434. (a)
1435. (c)	1436. (b)	1437. (a)	1438. (b)	1439. (d)	1440. (c)
1441. (c)	1442. (b)	1443. (a)	1444. (a)	1445. (b)	1446. (d)
1447. (d)	1448. (c)	1449. (a)	1450. (b)	1451. (d)	1452. (a)
1453. (d)	1454. (c)	1455. (c)	1456. (a)	1457. (d)	1458. (a)
1459. (d)	1460. (b)	1461. (d)	1462. (a)	1463. (d)	1464. (a)
1465. (a)	1466. (c)	1467. (b)	1468. (a)	1469. (c)	1470. (b)
1471. (a)	1472. (b)	1473. (d)	1474. (a)	1475. (d)	1476. (c)
1477. (d)	1478. (c)	1479. (b)	1480. (c)	1481. (c)	1482. (b)
1483. (b)	1484. (b)	1485. (d)	1486. (b)	1487. (a)	1488. (b)
1489. (a)	1490. (a)	1491. (b)	1492. (d)	1493. (d)	1494. (c)
1495. (b)	1496. (b)	1497. (a)	1498. (b)	1499. (b)	1500. (b)
1501. (a)	1502. (c)	1503. (d)	1504. (c)	1505. (d)	1506. (c)
1507. (d)	1508. (a)	1509. (b)	1510. (a)	1511. (b)	1512. (d)
1513. (c)	1514. (a)	1515. (b)	1516. (c)	1517. (d)	1518. (b)
1519. (a)	1520. (b)	1521. (a)	1522. (b)	1523. (c)	1524. (a)
1525. (c)	1526. (a)	1527. (b)	1528. (a)	1529. (d)	1530. (a)
1531. (b)	1532. (c)	1533. (d)	1534. (d)	1535. (b)	1536. (b)
1537. (a)	1538. (c)	1539. (d)	1540. (b)	1541. (b)	1542. (d)
1543. (a)	1544. (b)	1545. (d)	1546. (a)	1547. (c)	1548. (b)
1549. (d)	1550. (b)	1551. (d)	1552. (c)	1553. (a)	1554. (c)
1555. (a)	1556. (c)	1557. (b)	1558. (c)	1559. (b)	1560. (b)
1561. (b)	1562. (a)	1563. (c)	1564. (c)	1565. (d)	1566. (d)
1567. (b)	1568. (b)	1569. (a)	1570. (b)	1571. (a)	1572. (d)
1573. (a)	1574. (a)	1575. (b)	1576. (a)	1577. (c)	1578. (b)
1579. (c)	1580. (a)	1581. (b)	1582. (b)	1583. (d)	1584. (d)
1585. (b)	1586. (a)	1587. (c)	1588. (c)	1589. (d)	1590. (d)
1591. (b)	1592. (d)	1593. (b)	1594. (c)	1595. (c)	1596. (b)
1597. (b)	1598. (c)	1599. (c)	1600. (b)	1601. (a)	1602. (c)
1603. (a)	1604. (b)	1605. (c)	1606. (d)	1607. (a)	1608. (c)
1609. (c)	1610. (a)	1611. (c)	1612. (b)	1613. (c)	1614. (b)
1615. (c)	1616. (b)	1617. (d)	1618. (b)	1619. (c)	1620. (a)
1621. (b)	1622. (b)	1623. (b)	1624. (b)	1625. (a)	1626. (a)
1627. (a)	1628. (d)	1629. (a)	1630. (a)	1631. (b)	1632. (a)
1633. (b)	1634. (b)	1635. (d)	1636. (b)	1637. (d)	1638. (b)

Answers 209

1639. (c)	1640. (a)	1641. (a)	1642. (d)	1643. (b)	1644. (a)
1645. (c)	1646. (c)	1647. (c)	1648. (d)	1649. (c)	1650. (b)
1651. (b)	1652. (c)	1653. (b)	1654. (d)	1655. (b)	1656. (c)
1657. (b)	1658. (c)	1659. (d)	1660. (b)	1661. (b)	1662. (b)
1663. (a)	1664. (c)	1665. (c)	1666. (a)	1667. (a)	1668. (b)
1669. (b)	1670. (b)	1671. (c)	1672. (d)	1673. (b)	1674. (c)
1675. (d)	1676. (c)	1677. (c)	1678. (c)	1679. (c)	1680. (c)
1681. (c)	1682. (d)	1683. (b)	1684. (c)	1685. (d)	1686. (c)
1687. (c)	1688. (c)	1689. (d)	1690. (c)	1691. (d)	1692. (c)
1693. (a)	1694. (c)	1695. (a)	1696. (c)	1697. (b)	1698. (d)
1699. (d)	1700. (b)	1701. (a)	1702. (b)	1703. (b)	1704. (d)
1705. (c)	1706. (d)	1707. (a)	1708. (b)	1709. (d)	1710. (d)
1711. (c)	1712. (d)	1713. (c)	1714. (b)	1715. (a)	1716. (b)
1717. (b)	1718. (b)	1719. (a)	1720. (b)	1721. (a)	1722. (b)
1723. (a)	1724. (c)	1725. (a)	1726. (c)	1727. (d)	1728. (a)
1729. (c)	1730. (b)	1731. (a)	1732. (b)	1733. (b)	1734. (a)
1735. (c)	1736. (b)	1737. (a)	1738. (a)	1739. (b)	1740. (c)
1741. (a)	1742. (d)	1743. (a)	1744. (c)	1745. (d)	1746. (d)
1747. (a)	1748. (b)	1749. (c)	1750. (a)	1751. (b)	1752. (a)
1753. (b)	1754. (b)	1755. (b)	1756. (c)	1757. (c)	1758. (d)
1759. (d)	1760. (a)	1761. (b)	1762. (a)	1763. (b)	1764. (a)
1765. (c)	1766. (c)	1767. (d)	1768. (b)	1769. (a)	1770. (d)
1771. (b)	1772. (a)	1773. (a)	1774. (a)	1775. (a)	1776. (b)
1777. (d)	1778. (a)	1779. (d)	1780. (b)	1781. (b)	1782. (c)
1783. (d)	1784. (c)	1785. (b)	1786. (d)	1787. (d)	1788. (a)
1789. (b)	1790. (d)	1791. (d)	1792. (a)	1793. (c)	1794. (c)
1795. (d)	1796. (b)	1797. (a)	1798. (d)	1799. (a)	1800. (a)
1801. (b)	1802. (b)	1803. (a)	1804. (d)	1805. (b)	1806. (b)
1807. (c)	1808. (c)	1809. (c)	1810. (c)	1811. (c)	1812. (c)
1813. (b)	1814. (b)	1815. (a)	1816. (a)	1817. (c)	1818. (a)
1819. (a)	1820. (d)	1821. (b)	1822. (d)	1823. (b)	1824. (d)
1825. (b)	1826. (a)	1827. (b)	1828. (c)	1829. (d)	1830. (d)
1831. (b)	1832. (c)	1833. (c)	1834. (a)	1835. (a)	1836. (d)
1837. (a)	1838. (d)	1839. (c)	1840. (c)	1841. (d)	1842. (a)
1843. (d)	1844. (d)	1845. (a)	1846. (b)	1847. (c)	1848. (a)
1849. (c)	1850. (a)	1851. (d)	1852. (b)	1853. (a)	1854. (a)
1855. (d)	1856. (c)	1857. (a)	1858. (c)	1859. (b)	1860. (c)
1861. (d)	1862. (b)	1863. (c)	1864. (c)	1865. (c)	1866. (b)
1867. (b)	1868. (d)	1869. (a)	1870. (b)	1871. (d)	1872. (b)

1873. (d) 1874. (a) 1875. (d) 1876. (a) 1877. (b) 1878. (a)
1879. (d) 1880. (c) 1881. (a) 1882. (a) 1883. (d) 1884. (b)
1885. (b) 1886. (c)

CHAPTER X : SPECIAL SENSES

1887. (a) 1888. (d) 1889. (b) 1890. (a) 1891. (b) 1892. (a)
1893. (d) 1894. (c) 1895. (a) 1896. (b) 1897. (a) 1898. (
1899. (b) 1900. (d) 1901. (a) 1902. (a) 1903. (d) 1904. (
1905. (d) 1906. (d) 1907. (b) 1908. (b) 1909. (d) 1910. (
1911. (c) 1912. (d) 1913. (a) 1914. (c) 1915. (a) 1916. (
1917. (a) 1918. (a) 1919. (b) 1920. (b) 1921. (a) 1922. (
1923. (d) 1924. (d) 1925. (a) 1926. (c) 1927. (b) 1928. (
1929. (a) 1930. (c) 1931. (a) 1932. (a) 1933. (b) 1934. (
1935. (b) 1936. (a) 1937. (c) 1938. (a) 1939. (b) 1940. (
1941. (a) 1942. (b) 1943. (a) 1944. (a) 1945. (b) 1946. (
1947. (a) 1948. (b) 1949. (a) 1950. (c) 1951. (b) 1952. (
1953. (d) 1954. (a) 1955. (d) 1956. (a) 1957. (a) 1958. (
1959. (c) 1960. (c) 1961. (a) 1962. (c) 1963. (c) 1964. (
1965. (a) 1966. (b) 1967. (b) 1968. (a) 1969. (d) 1970. (
1971. (c) 1972. (a) 1973. (a) 1974. (b) 1975. (c) 1976. (
1977. (c) 1978. (b) 1979. (a) 1980. (a) 1981. (a) 1982. (
1983. (a) 1984. (a) 1985. (a) 1986. (a) 1987. (c) 1988. (
1989. (b) 1990. (b) 1991. (d) 1992. (c) 1993. (d) 1994. (
1995. (d) 1996. (a) 1997. (c) 1998. (d)

CHAPTER XI : RADIOLOGY AND IMAGING METHODS

1999. (b) 2000. (a) 2001. (d) 2002. (d) 2003. (d) 2004. (
2005. (a) 2006. (d) 2007. (b) 2008. (a) 2009. (b) 2010. (
2011. (c) 2012. (b) 2013. (a) 2014. (b) 2015. (a) 2016. (
2017. (d) 2018. (d) 2019. (b) 2020. (a) 2021. (a) 2022. (
2023. (c) 2024. (c) 2025. (a) 2026. (b) 2027. (b) 2028. (
2029. (a) 2030. (c) 2031. (d) 2032. (b) 2033. (a) 2034. (
2035. (a) 2036. (c)

References

1. Gray's Anatomy - Williams, Warwick et al., 38th edition.
2. Clinically Oriented Anatomy - Keith L. Moore.
3. Applied Anatomy - R.J. Last.
4. The Developing Human - Keith L. Moore.
5. Human Embryology - Hamilton, Boyd and Mossmans.
6. Emery's Elements of Medical Genetics - Muller, Young, 9th edition.
7. Human Genetics - Gangane.
8. Genetics in Medicine - Thomson and Thomson.
9. Textbook of Histology - I.B. Singh.
10. Journal of Applied Medicine, May 1993, page 385-392. Guide to Postgraduate Exams - Multiple Choice Questions - Garesh J. Holsgrove.
11. The Art of Teaching Medical Students - MET Cell, Seth, G.S. Medical College - Joglekar, Bhuiyan.
12. The Medical Teacher, Edinburgh, Churchill Livingstone, 1982. "How to Construct a Fair Multiple Choice Question Paper', Cox, K.R., Ewance.
13. Indian Journal of Medical Education 186, 'Formative Evaluation of Undergraduate Students by MCQ Tests' - Shah, K.U., Kulkarni, S.D.
14. Pre-PG Test Review - Third Ed., 1990, G. Omkarnath.
15. Medicines New Vision - National Geographic, Jan. 1987, pp. 4-40.
16. Langman's Medical Embryology, Sixth ed., Saddler, T.W.